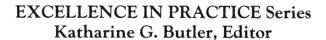

EXCELLENCE IN PRACTICE Series
Katharine G. Butler, Editor

FAMILY–CENTERED EARLY INTERVENTION FOR COMMUNICATION DISORDERS

Prevention and Treatment

EXCELLENCE IN PRACTICE Series
Katharine G. Butler, Editor

Conversational Management with Language–Impaired Children
Bonnie Brinton and Martin Fujuki

Successful Interactive Skills for Speech–Language
Pathologists and Audiologists
Dorothy Molyneaux and Vera W. Lane

Communicating for Learning: Classroom Observation
and Collaboration
Elaine R. Silliman and Louise Cherry Wilkinson

Hispanic Children and Adults with Communication Disorders:
Assessment and Prevention
Henriette W. Langdon with Li–Rong Lilly Cheng

Family–Centered Early Intervention for Communication Disorders:
Prevention and Treatment
Gail Donahue–Kilburg

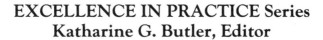

EXCELLENCE IN PRACTICE Series
Katharine G. Butler, Editor

FAMILY–CENTERED EARLY INTERVENTION FOR COMMUNICATION DISORDERS

Prevention and Treatment

Gail Donahue–Kilburg, PhD
Associate Professor
Communication Sciences and Disorders
Towson State University
Towson, Maryland

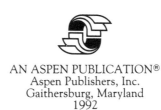

AN ASPEN PUBLICATION®
Aspen Publishers, Inc.
Gaithersburg, Maryland
1992

Library of Congress Cataloging-in-Publication Data

Donahue-Kilburg, Gail.
Family-centered early intervention for communication disorders :
prevention and treatment / Gail Donahue-Kilburg
p.   cm. — (Excellence in practice series)

Includes bibliographical references and index.
ISBN: 0-8342-0294-8
1. Communicative disorders in children — Prevention.
2. Communicative disorders in children — Treatment.
3. Communicative disorders in children — Patients — Family relationships.
I. Title.   II. Series
RJ496.C67D66   1992
618.92'85505—dc20
92-4705
CIP

Editorial Services: Ruth Bloom

Library of Congress Catalog Card Number: 92-4705
ISBN: 0-8342-0294-8

Printed in the United States of America

1 2 3 4 5

To my family—
nuclear, extended, and selected

Table of Contents

Series Foreword

"It's Just Talking, Isn't it?"

Nowhere in the field of speech-language pathology and audiology is there greater need to address *preventive intervention* than within the early years of infancy and toddlerhood. The passage of Public Law 94-142 in the 1980s has galvanized the health and educational systems of this country to address very young children's needs in new and creative ways. Donahue-Kilburg describes a number of these new approaches in this book. In this very accessible rendition of current approaches, she assist not only speech-language pathologists and audiologists to capture the essence of service delivery in emerging arena of early intervention. Consonant with current legislation, the author details how the family and communication development intertwine, providing the nexus for understanding how it is that the family context can be used to assess and intervene with the very young.

Implicit in the early chapters of the book is the evidence developed from research over the past two or three decades in how infant abilities develop through early schemas. Cognitive development stems from the hearing, looking, sucking and grasping that infants undertake. The literature in child development has shown how *before* and *at* birth, the infants are capable of discriminating variations in human speech (Aslin, Pisoni & Jusczyk, 1983; Columbo, 1986). The visual system, as well as the auditory system, is more highly developed than previously thought, with children in the very weeks of life developing a preference for faces over objects (Vandenberg, 1991). The social capabilities are revealed through reactive crying. In fact, it is the social nature of even the young infant that has led to the realization that the family context in which this infant is born and reared will mark the child's growth and development. As Vandenburg (1991) maintains "the infant is biologically anchored and oriented in the social world. The adaptive utility of this is apparent, given how helplessly dependent infants are on their caretakers" (p. 1282). In fact, the infants' sense of attunement to, and attachment with, caregivers is thought by some (Stern, 1985) to provide the opportunity for infants to develop a core self with others, i.e., the caregivers in the immediate environment. These are the assumptions that underlie the framework by which Donahue-Kilburg builds the case for the importance of the family unit.

As Gebbs and Teti (1990) have noted:

> the field of . . . early intervention has grown dramatically . . . broadening from a focus on the child's cognitive and motor abilities to a focus on the whole child in the context of his or her family and social environment. This expansion has brought professionals to-gether in an effort to develop useful methods of assessing the strengths and needs of infants and their families. (p. 317)

It is to this end that Donahue-Kilburg has brought her rich background and experience to bear. While designed to meet the assessment and intervention needs of those professionals in communicative disorders, the text has much to offer to the transdisciplinary and multidisciplinary terms of professionals in growing field of early intervention. The importance of communication, whether it be verbal or nonverbal, stands at the center of the human condition. As such, its worth cannot be overestimated. That it is frequently underestimated was reflected in a graduate student's comment to me regarding infant and toddler language acquisition and disorders during a recent course I was teaching. The class was composed of special educators, psychologists, nurses, occupational and physical therapists, speech-language pathologists, audiologists, teachers of the deaf, social workers, and even a parent or two. Given the varying perspectives, the instructor had spent considerable time tracing the course of early communication, particularly that which occurs (or does not occur) between caregivers and very young children. One student commented to the group at large, "I don't know what's so important about this. It's just grown-ups talking, isn't it?"

As those reading this text will ratify, communication and its disorders is not related to "just talking." We have Dr. Donahue-Kilburg to thank for making it clear that there is much more than just talking occurring in the tapestry that goes into the make up of the child-family context.

KATHARINE G. BUTLER, PhD
Series Editor
Excellence in Practice Series
Syracuse University
Syracuse, New York

REFERENCES

Aslin, R.N., Pisoni, D.B., & Jusczyk. (1983). Auditory development and speech perception in infancy. In M.M. Haith & J.J. Campos (Eds.) *Handbook of child psychology: Vol. 2. Infancy and development psychology* (pp. 573–688). New York: John Wiley & Sons.

Gebbi, E.D., & Teti, D.M. (1990). *Interdisciplinary Assessment of Infants: A Guide for Early Intervention Professionals.* Baltimore: Paul H. Brookes.

Stern, D. (1985). *The impersonal world of the infant.* New York: Basic Books.

Vandenberg, G. (1991). Is epistemology enough? An essential consideration of development. *American Psychologist, 46*:12, December, 1278–1286.

Preface

The past few years have seen an explosion of information concerning early psychosocial development, parent-child interaction, infant/toddler communication development, changing family structure and function, and the interaction of all of these factors. At the same time, professionals have come to believe that any effort to provide therapeutic services to infants and toddlers who are at risk for developmental problems must involve the children's families. The movement to create early intervention services that are sensitive to family needs and characteristics has been spurred on by the passage of the federal law, P.L. 99-457, that provides incentives for states to develop family-centered services.

In the midst of these changes in information and service delivery systems, professionals are rethinking their interactions with families. Clinicians who were educated to provide more traditional services that did not involve families in planning and delivering treatment services are trying new ways of working collaboratively with families and other professionals. Students who are preparing for clinical work are faced with assimilating the wide variety of literature on families, communication development, and treatment methodologies that are appropriate for infants, toddlers, and their families.

Family-Centered Early Intervention for Communication Disorders is designed to provide a broad range of information on family structure and function in our multicultural society, family system characteristics and the implications for intervention, communication development in the family context, the nature and devliery of family-centered services, the requirements of P.L. 99-457, and the competencies that such services require, as well as ways to approach planning, assessment, and treatment that involve families in practical ways. It is written for students and practicing clinicians who are especially interested in helping families to promote communication development in their infants and toddlers who may have impairments that put development at risk.

I have divided the book into three parts. Part I, the Family and Communication Development, considers the role that the family plays as a context for communication development for both normally developing and communication disordered children. Part II, Preventive Intervention in the Family Context, provides a general overview of family-centered intervention, information on the impact of P.L. 99-457, and skills the clinician needs for working with families. The final section, Part III, Preventive Intervention in the Family Context: Assessment and Intervention, fives ideas for evaluating the family in general and as a context for communication development, for evaluating the child as a communicator, and strategies for planning and carrying out effective information with young children and their families.

Some of the more theoretical chapters contain exercises designed to help the reader process and integrate the information. Many of these exercises would also work well as classroom activities. The chapters on assessment and intervention have appendixes that contain a case study to illustrate the application of the ideas presented in the chapters, as well as other materials such as example IFSP forms, forms for clinical use in assessment and intervention, and a family-centered service assessment tool.

Gail Donahue-Kilburg

Acknowledgments

Many people helped me to learn, gather, and assemble the information in this book. Others provided support, time, encouragement, suggestions, criticism, or a peaceful place to write. Still others gently pushed me when I needed it or helped me laugh and start over when I got to what seemed like an impass in writing or living. Thank you all.

I especially thank the families and professionals I have worked with in Pennsylvania, Vermont, Maryland, and Maine. I have learned from them all. My colleagues and students at Towson State University also deserve my gratitude for encouragement, support, and information. I am particularly grateful for the assigned time grants, research grants, and sabbatical leave which were supported or provided by Dr. Bill Wallace, the Faculty Research Committee, Dean Steven Collier, and the Sabbatical Leave Committee.

My professional colleagues and friends in the area of infant-toddler intervention have given many good suggestions and helped me to find information. I'd like to give special thanks to: Shirley Sparks, Margaret Briggs, Ayala Manolson, Camille Cattlet, Debra Reichert Hoge, and Candace Warner.

Barry Guitar was instrumental in helping me develop some of the techniques for working with families. In addition, he also read and commented on some of the early attempts to organize the information. His help has been most valuable.

The librarians at the Patten Free Library in Bath, Maine, have been helpful and willing to find and obtain many obscure volumes. Their help made the final revisions possible.

The illustrator of this book, Gethyn L. Bridgeman, is a wonder. Her visual interpretation of the words was done quickly and with very little guidance from me.

I'd like to thank Richard Kilburg for encouragement and some helpful comments on the first chapters. Ben Kilburg, our son, deserves a greater deal of credit for my involvement in early intervention and family-centered practice. Thank you, Ben, for that and for the inspiration to do what I believe in.

The people at Aspen have been a pleasure to work with. Loretta Stock has been particularly supportive, and Kay Butler has provided many helpful suggestions for improvements to the manuscript.

Finally, the support of some people has been invaluable at various stages of this project. I owe special thanks to Michele Barattucci, Barbara and Charlie Nardozzi, and to my parents, Bill and Gerry Donahue. This book might never have been finished without the laughter, caring, and fresh approach to life that Gerry Pepin has helped me find. Thank you, Gerry.

Part I

The Family and Communication Development

The first section of this book considers the role that the family plays as a context for communication development for both normally developing and communication-disordered children.

1

The Family Context

One television network's evening news program runs a standard feature called "The American Family." A weekly news magazine has recently published an entire special issue on the changes in families and family life. The American family is big news.

At the same time, the family is being recognized as a potent force in child development. The family is being called upon to use its influence to promote the best possible development of all its members. As a society, we focus on the development of not only our strong and healthy family members who will grow up to be track stars and merit scholars, but also on members for whom it will be more difficult to excel or even to develop necessary skills. The media coverage of the widespread effects on infants of maternal drug and alcohol abuse, AIDS, and poverty has helped to focus society's attention on children with problems and on their families. There is now more public attention given to children who begin life with some condition that creates a developmental risk and on those who, after an apparently normal beginning, experience unexpected problems.

Nowhere is the importance of the family felt more strongly than in the field of early intervention. The war on poverty and the civil rights movement of the 1960s and 1970s fostered an enhanced societal belief in the right of every individual to have an equal opportunity to become educated and to lead a fulfilling life. This belief, coupled with a growing body of information on an infant's ability to learn and to benefit from positive early experiences, has increased society's belief in and demand for early education programs for children with problems. Early preventive intervention that begins soon after the identification of an impairment or risk factor—often in early infancy—has become a right of children in most states.

The family has become an important focus in early intervention efforts because experience and research have shown that optimal infant/toddler development can only be promoted within the family context. The importance of this family focus is emphasized by Public Law 99-457, passed by Congress in 1986, which addresses the need for services to high-risk and handicapped infants and

3

toddlers. The law calls for "family-centered" services for this population and underscores our growing national awareness of the family's role in early intervention.

This book is written by a speech-language clinician for people who are, or will soon become, speech-language clinicians working with infants, toddlers, and their families. It is also addressed to practitioners and students in other professions, such as audiology, who are primarily concerned with the communication abilities and development of very young children. It is the author's belief that effective clinical work with infants and toddlers requires an understanding of the family and its role in early development. Therefore, to provide quality family-centered services, professionals must have some basic knowledge of the family in general as well as a framework for considering the unique characteristics of specific families.

Despite clinicians' sincere belief in the importance of the family, few of us know much about the family—its nature or function—beyond our own experiences as family members. This chapter summarizes some current views of the American family, its nature, functions, development, and variations.

THE NATURE OF THE FAMILY

Most practitioners bring certain ideas of what a family is to their clinical interactions. These ideas may be largely based on personal experiences with Mom, Dad, and siblings or with other families we've known intimately, such as the family in the next apartment or the families of our best friends when we were children or adolescents. It's also based on families we've read about or seen on television. The Cunninghams of "Happy Days" fame and Bill Cosby's Huxtables have probably etched new family possibilities and expectations onto many of our experience-based ideas of what a family is.

For many people, clinicians included, the family is a group of people brought together by marriage or birth; it includes a mother, a father, and one or more children. We are aware, however, of many variations on this theme. There are, for example, the single-parent family, the blended family made up of parents (one or both of whom have been previously married) and their children from both the previous and current marriages, the multigenerational family, the family of two gay or lesbian partners and their adopted child or children, and the family in which the parents are not legally married to each other. These configurations of families may have come to fit easily, or not so easily, into our conception of what a family is, especially as it relates to the needs of a young child. But our idea of the family must also include the foster families that may fulfill the caregiver role for some of our young clients, as well as the institutions, such as day care centers and orphanages, that provide care for some

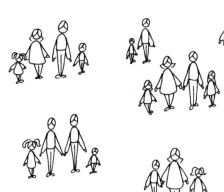

infants and toddlers. Also, our idea of a family must be sensitive to cultural and socioeconomic variations in family structure and function.

The literature from a number of different disciplines, such as sociology and psychology, suggests definitions of the family that might be useful as guides for our consideration of the family. Some of these definitions fit the traditional, middle-class family of the 1950s better than they do the changing and varied family structures that we are aware of today. For example, Reiss (1971) argues that the universal aspect of the family is ". . . a small kinship-structured group with the key function of nurturant socialization of the newborn" (p. 19). More specifically, Goode (1982) lists the following relationships that constitute a family:

1. At least two adult persons of opposite sex live together
2. They engage in some form of division of labor; that is—they do not both perform exactly the same tasks
3. They engage in economic, social, and emotional exchanges, that is, they do things for each other
4. They share many things in common, such as food, sex, residence, and both goods and social activities
5. The adults have parental relations with their children, as their children have filial relations with them; the parents have some authority over their children and both share with one another while also assuming some obligation for protection, cooperation, and nurturance.
6. There are sibling relations among the children themselves with, once more, a range of obligations to share, protect, and help one another. (p. 9)

While Reiss' and Goode's definitions shed light on the nature of the family, neither of them encompasses all of the examples of possible family structures listed earlier. We need a less restrictive definition to fit the wide range of traditional and nontraditional families we see today. For example, Kenkel (1977) considers the family ". . . a dynamic, semi-closed system of interacting personalities" (p. 442). He sees the family as *dynamic* because it is characterized by activity, change, and movement, as *semi-closed* because it responds to changes in other systems, and as a *system* because each position or role in the family is related to each other position in the family. As one member of the family changes, the whole family system changes.

Kenkel's definition introduces the important concept of the family as a system. A system, according to Merriam-Webster (1974), is a "group of units so combined as to form a whole and to operate in unison" (p. 694). Several authors (e.g., Bowen [1978], Minuchin [1974], Satir [1972]) have envisioned the family as a human system with people as its units and each person's "operations" affecting every other person in the system. This idea will be explored in greater detail later.

In addition to this systems-based idea of what a family is, it may help to remember that the nuclear family (Mom, Dad, and the children) may not be the only unit that we need to consider clinically. We may also become involved with the extended family and what could be called the "selected" family. The extended family includes grandparents and other members of the kinship structure who may often be powerful influences on the nuclear family. The selected family includes close friends and other persons, such as teachers, mentors, or social group leaders (e.g., the tribal shaman), who may at times fulfill the functions of family members.

A definition of the family is only useful to us as clinicians if it helps us to identify the people who influence and support the family member(s) with whom we work. If the definition is too restricted, we may fail to identify important people; if it is too broad, we may waste time considering people who play little or no role in the day-to-day functioning of the family.

EXERCISE #1

Stop reading for a few minutes and think about your own family. Who are the members of your nuclear family? List these people in the spaces below:

_____   _____   _____

_____   _____   _____

Now consider your extended family and/or your selected family. On the lines below list people from these parts of your family who should be considered by a professional working with you in your family context. Include any people who are strong influences on your behavior or beliefs as well as people who provide a significant amount of support (emotional or otherwise) for you.

_____   _____   _____

_____   _____   _____

FUNCTIONS OF THE FAMILY

"What each family member is and what each will become is, to some extent, affected by the family group to which he belongs" (Kenkel, 1977, p. 443). This statement illustrates the great influence of the family on individual development, an influence that is largely based on the functions the family performs for society. In most societies the family is charged with the functions of (1) child bearing and the establishment of legal responsibility for the child, (2) child rearing—providing food, clothing, and protection, (3) socialization—passing on the skills, norms, and values of the culture or subculture including its language, attitudes, beliefs, and patterns of behavior, and (4) regulation of sexual behavior (Nock, 1987; Kenkel, 1977). In essence, the family is to provide the setting, goods, and relationships which should make people competent, comfortable members of society.

Satir (1972, 1988) thinks of the family as a factory where people are made, and of parents as "peoplemakers." She sees the family as providing self-worth, communication, rules, and a link to society. These factors are dealt with differently in each family. Some families are "nurturing" families in which members experience (1) high self-worth, (2) direct, clear, specific, and honest communication, (3) flexible, human, appropriate, and changeable rules, and (4) an open and hopeful link to society. Other families are "troubled" and their members experience (1) low self-worth, (2) indirect, vague, or dishonest communication, (3) rigid, inhuman, and non-negotiable rules, and (4) a fearful, placating, or blaming link to society (Satir, 1972). In reality, all families exist on a continuum somewhere between nurturing and troubled, and probably change position on that continuum frequently.

Satir's conception of families as nurturing or troubled is much like the recently popular idea of "functional" versus "dysfunctional" families. In functional families, every member performs his or her roles and relates to each other family member in a healthy, supportive way most of the time. Children are expected and allowed to be children—imperfect, dependent, and immature. The family is consequently able to perform its functions for society in that the children are nurtured, socialized, etc. (Bradshaw, 1988; Mellody, Miller, & Miller, 1989).

Families in which the parents do not meet the needs of the children are dysfunctional families. Parents in such families are often needy people who have come from troubled families. Such parents are unable to model healthy self-esteem or caregiving for their children. Instead, they often cast their children in the role of caregivers who must meet their parents' needs. In dysfunctional families, one or more persons are often addicted to some chemical, work, food, etc. (Bradshaw, 1988; Mellody et al., 1989).

The family has a big job to do for every child born or accepted into it, regardless of that child's risk or health status. Some families have the resources and abilities to do the job fairly well, and others need a great deal of help and support if they are to develop those capacities.

DEVELOPMENT OF THE FAMILY

Traditionally, a family is created when two young, childless adults are married (we can set the variations on this theme aside for the time being). This nascent family does not become magically endowed with the ability to carry out all of the functions of a family with the simple act of exchanging wedding vows. The individual members and the family system develop their roles and abilities over time.

Several sociological concepts are helpful to the understanding of family development. These include: family positions, family roles, family life cycle, and developmental tasks. All of these concepts figure in the Family Development approach to studying the family. This conceptual framework draws on the work of Duvall (1971), Rodgers (1962), and Havighurst (1952), and has been synthesized by Kenkel (1977). Understanding these concepts can help clinicians to sensitively assess and counsel families of children in need of early intervention.

From its inception, each traditional nuclear family has positions (Rodgers, 1962). In the beginning there are just two positions, the "wife" and the "husband."

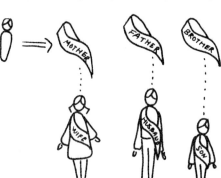

As family members are added, new positions develop. For example, with the birth of a female child the position "daughter" is added, and the previously existing positions change to "wife-mother" and "husband-father." With the birth of a second child, the daughter position also changes to "daughter-sister."

Each position in a family has certain behavioral expectations, or function-related roles, attached to it. For example, the position of wife-mother may be associated with roles such as caregiver, cook, chauffeur, laundress, lover, wage earner, nurse, money manager, disciplinarian, friend, housekeeper, general manager, mediator, and advocate. The roles that go with each family position are called its "role cluster" and the role clusters of all family members added together make up the "role complex" of the family (Rodgers, 1962). The role cluster of each family member is negotiated and develops over time; the family role complex changes with every new position added or existing position removed (Kenkel, 1977; Nock, 1987).

EXERCISE #2

Think about the positions and functional roles in your family system. In the chart below, fill in the positions and role clusters that make up your family's role complex. Chart a role cluster for each person that you listed in Exercise #1.

Family System—Role Complex

POSITIONS	*ROLE CLUSTERS*	
Name _____	_____	_____
Position_____	_____	_____
_____	_____	_____
_____	_____	_____
	* * *	
Name _____	_____	_____
Position_____	_____	_____
_____	_____	_____
_____	_____	_____
	* * *	
Name _____	_____	_____
Position_____	_____	_____
_____	_____	_____
_____	_____	_____
	* * *	
Name _____	_____	_____
Position_____	_____	_____
_____	_____	_____
_____	_____	_____

(Please use additional sheets if necessary.)

The ideas of family positions and roles are important to the concept of family life cycle. Families have a life cycle much like that of an individual human being. Families begin, grow, develop, and eventually cease to exist with the death or departure of their members (Kenkel, 1977). The family life cycle progresses as the family positions change, as family members' role clusters change, and as these role changes affect the family role complex.

It is with the idea of family life cycle that the concept of the family as a system of interdependent, mutually influential members becomes especially clear. As each family member grows and develops or changes in some less-than-positive way (e.g., becomes ill or fails to develop), his or her role in the family changes, and as individual roles change, the family role complex changes.

The family enters a new stage of life cycle every time its role complex changes (Kenkel, 1977). Conversely, "each shift in family life cycle status demands a readjustment in every aspect of the roles of all family members" (Kenkel, 1966, p. 395). For example, when an infant begins to walk, her role in the family changes slightly. She had been a person who could be expected to move fairly slowly from one place to another and to explore only those things from floor level to about 18 inches above the floor. In response to this expectation, other family members could play the role of caregiver and guardian for this child from a relatively stationary position and not worry too much about breakable or inedible articles that were not directly on the floor with the child. One could think of this as playing the role of the seated, relaxed, minimally vigilant guardian near whom the infant could usually be trusted to stay. With the advent of walking and the child's desire to practice this skill over broad reaches of terrain, these roles and the relationship change. The child, who has become a toddler, can be expected to move quickly from one place to another, even out of the room where the caregiver is seated, and to investigate anything in reach from her new, upright position. No longer can the caregiver be stationary or minimally vigilant. The caregiver's role becomes that of follower or chaser who frequently, in the nontoddler-proofed house, has to fish inedible objects out of the child's mouth or clean up spilled or broken items. The caregiver's role has changed to mobile, highly vigilant guardian. Others in the family will also adjust to the changes in both the infant and the caregiver. The infant's acquisition of a new skill changed her role, her caregivers' roles, and promoted the family to the next substage in the family life cycle, from "family with infant" to "family with toddler." The system shifted in response to the developmental change in the child.

There are some important factors that influence a family's progress from one stage to another. Duvall (1971) lists four criteria for life cycle stages: (1) presence or absence of children; (2) age of the oldest child; (3) grade in school of the oldest child; and (4) a combination of age, occupation, and status factors of the couple. Duvall (1985) also has delineated eight major stages of the family life cycle which result from the interaction of these factors

Stage 1—Married Couples (without children)
Stage 2—Childbearing Families (oldest child 0 to 30 months)
Stage 3—Families with Preschool Children (oldest child 2.5 to 6 years)
Stage 4—Families with School Children (oldest child 6 to 13 years)
Stage 5—Families with Teenagers (oldest child 13 to 20 years)
Stage 6—Families as Launching Centers (first child gone to last leaving home)
Stage 7—Families in Middle Years (empty nest to retirement)
Stage 8—Aging Families (retirement to death of one or both)
(pp. 116-117)

Duvall's stages need some reconsideration. For example, we might change married couples to "committed couples," and we might consider adding some optional life cycle stages such as "families in which the parents are separated or divorced," "families in middle years with adult children who never leave or return home," or "families in middle years who have primary responsibility for raising grandchildren."

Whatever the list of family life cycle stages we may find useful, the transition to each stage is brought about by changes in one or more family member(s) and necessitates changes in all other members. In this way the family truly works like a system, with change in one part bringing about change in all of the others. Satir (1972) envisions this system as a mobile on which all family members are delicately balanced. If you shift the position of one family mobile figure, all of the other figures are out of balance until they too shift positions.

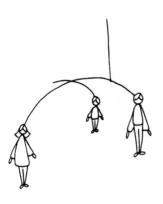
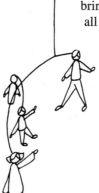

EXERCISE #3

Again, stop and consider your own family's status. In what stage of the family life cycle is your family now?

What event(s) or changes placed the family in that stage?

What adjustments were required of family members when that change occurred?

The notion of developmental tasks can shed further light on the changing identity and function of the family. Havighurst (1952) defines a developmental task as ". . . a task which arises at or about a certain period in the life of the individual and successful achievement of which leads to his happiness and to success with later tasks, while failure leads to unhappiness in the individual, disapproval by society, and difficulty with later tasks" (p. 2). These tasks can be grouped into three broad categories: (1) physical abilities (e.g., learning to walk), (2) mental skills (e.g., learning arithmetic), and (3) attitudes (e.g., trust) (Kenkel, 1977; Nock, 1987). The accomplishment of a developmental task is not necessarily an all-or-none or now-or-never proposition. We may partially gain the skills or abilities at the appropriate developmental time, and we may do further work toward completion of the task later in life.

This concept of developmental tasks also helps in our understanding of the family as a system. As Kenkel (1977) states:

> Each family member can be viewed as an individual striving to accomplish certain developmental tasks while interacting with other individuals. No family member can be viewed in absolute isolation. . . . Knowing the developmental demands placed on family members at the different stages of the life cycle of a group allows us to evaluate the family in a relative rather than an absolute manner. The better equipped a family is for each of its members to meet his developmental tasks and the closer each comes to accomplishing them, the more successful is the family. (p. 455)

All family members have developmental tasks to accomplish. For example, the newly married pair must learn to communicate effectively, achieve a satisfactory sexual relationship, and learn to resolve conflicts (to list but a few of their tasks). When children are born, tasks are added. The new parents must (1) develop a philosophy of child rearing, (2) develop caregiving skills, and (3) provide food, shelter, and clothing, while still trying to develop as human beings (Kenkel, 1977).

There are also many developmental tasks for the children to master. These tasks fall into the categories of health, intelligence, empathy, autonomy, judgment, and creativity. During infancy and early childhood, children must learn to eat solid foods, to walk, and to gain bladder and bowel control. They must learn to talk, develop concepts, learn to trust, love, and share, learn to be away from their parents, and to accept responsibility for tasks such as dressing. And they must learn how, when, where, and with whom to play. They must begin to make choices and learn to deal with changes in routine (Kenkel, 1977). These are only a few examples of developmental tasks of childhood.

The ideas of family life cycle and developmental tasks emphasize the ongoing changes that take place in family life. Change, whether it is positive or negative, is almost always accompanied by some degree of stress. With each addition or subtraction of a family member and each family member role change, the family will experience some stress. In addition, all family members progress toward the mastery of their developmental tasks while they are interacting with other family members who are also working on their own developmental tasks. When the tasks are complementary, the changes are probably perceived as positive by everyone involved. When the tasks are not complementary, additional stress may result from the changes and interactions.

EXERCISE #4

What are your current developmental tasks? (The broad categories include physical abilities, mental skills, and attitudes.)

_____

_____

Do they complement those of other members of your family, or are your sets of tasks likely to create some conflict?

_____

_____

The previous discussion of family positions, roles, and tasks presents families as though they are all reasonably nurturing/functional with each member fulfilling his or her roles in a capable manner. This is not always true, and many clinicians will work with families who are troubled/dysfunctional. With those families, it may be helpful to expand the idea of roles. In addition to function-related roles, family members can be seen as having emotional/psychological roles to play in the family system. These emotional/psychological roles are related to fulfillment of the family's basic needs. According to Bradshaw (1988), each family needs "a sense of worth, a sense of physical security or productivity, a sense of intimacy and relatedness, a sense of unified structure, a sense of responsibility, a need for challenge and stimulation, a sense of joy and affirmation and a spiritual grounding" (p. 31). If the people who fill the parent positions in the family don't provide the family with these basic needs, other family members will do so by filling emotional/psychological roles such as "hero," "superachiever," "Mom's buddy," "peacemaker," "family scapegoat," or "clown" (Bradshaw, 1988).

In dysfunctional family systems, family members who take on these roles may lose their own true identity and get stuck in the emotional/psychological roles more or less permanently. Trying to change roles causes a great deal of upheaval in the dysfunctional family system. In healthy, functional family systems the roles are less rigid. Different family members can take different roles at various times because the roles are flexible and rotating (Bradshaw, 1988).

The current popular literature is full of reports on the damage that occurs when a family member sacrifices his or her identity to fill an emotional/psychological role for the family. The condition which results is referred to as "codependence," and it is considered to be a psychiatric disease entity which is characterized by difficulties with self-esteem, interpersonal boundaries, identity, experiencing personal needs and wants, and experiencing and doing things in moderation (Mellody et al., 1989). These concepts are important to our more complete understanding of the families with whom we work.

All of the family structure and development concepts that have been discussed can be used to gain a better understanding of families and the ways in which they function in society. They can also shed light on the operation of a specific family. It is easier to understand and empathize with a family's inability to carry out a treatment plan for a developmentally delayed 2-year-old child, for example, if the clinician knows that the family is experiencing a great deal of stress because a grandparent has just moved into the family home, an older sibling has recently started school, and the father has taken on an additional part-time job. All of these changes require adaptation and adjustment by all family members, and adaptation takes energy. When such changes are underway, there may not be enough energy to deal with all of the day-to-day demands of the family routine.

The next section explores the ways parents develop their abilities to provide care for and to socialize their children. Their development of parenting and socialization practices seems especially important to the understanding of the family as a context for communication growth.

THE DEVELOPMENT OF PARENTING/SOCIALIZATION PRACTICES

Parents set the tone for family function and interaction. Their growth into their roles as parents and their development of parenting skills is of prime importance to the eventual functioning of the family. Alvy (1981) views parenting ". . . as consisting of several inter-related functions and responsibilities. These are (1) providing resources to maintain family and home, (2) caring for the home, (3) protecting children, (4) the physical and psychological caregiving of children, and (5) advocating for children and interfacing with the community and wider society" (p. 1). Among these functions, the physical and psychological caregiving of children seems especially relevant to communication growth. This entails all of the physical and psychological techniques and skills the parents may acquire to promote the child's development of social, emotional, cognitive, motor, and linguistic abilities. These are, essentially, the parents' caregiving or child-rearing techniques. Whether consciously or unconsciously, the parents must develop a philosophy of child rearing and the skills to enact that philosophy. How parents accomplish these things is one of the major issues of parenting.

Many factors influence new parents as they begin to fashion their child-rearing philosophy and behaviors. Among these influences are hormonal and instinctual factors, family example and experience, societal influences transmitted by the media, and even some information learned from "experts" via books, videos, or formal coursework. According to Westby (1987), child-rearing practices are affected by "the perceived capability of infants and the culture's goals for children's development, the intentionality of infants, and infants' susceptibility to supernatural harm" (p. 11). The practices that eventually evolve probably result from the interaction of education, personality, coping ability, behaviors of the child, stress, maturity, developmental task priorities, cultural beliefs, and environmental pressures.

Satir (1972, 1988) considers this process as coming up with family "blueprints" for "peoplemaking" and points out that it's easiest to duplicate your own parents' blueprints. This duplication is often an unconscious process; parents simply do with their children what they remember having done with them as children. While this may often have a positive outcome, it also has been blamed for the continuation of such practices as child abuse in successive generations of some families. It is also common, and usually more conscious, for new parents to reject their parents' child-rearing practices and to try to do things differently. "Unfortunately, deciding what not to do is not the whole story. You have to decide what you are going to do and how you are going to do it" (Satir, 1972, p. 200).

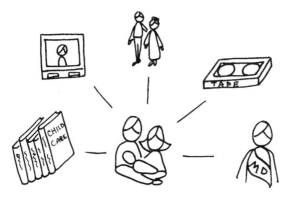

To develop their own philosophy of child rearing, a couple may choose to put more emphasis on individual development or on conformity to societal expectations. They may also determine some personality goals for the child (e.g., outgoing, fearless) or some basic orientation to child rearing (e.g., set an example to be emulated, refrain from physical punishment) (Kenkel, 1977). Whatever the conscious philosophy, the child-rearing practices develop in response to many of the variables noted above. The couple's own parents' blueprint may sometimes take over when they least expect it; societal influences and the child's characteristics may exert strong pressures for the parents to react in certain ways.

The new parents' philosophy and practices develop during a stage of "transition to parenthood" which occurs when the first child is born (Nock, 1987; Vincent, 1979). During this time, the couple makes the transition from dyad to triad, and unfortunately child-rearing practices are but one concern during this transition. There is a reported drop in satisfaction with the married couples' relationship after the birth of the first child (Vincent, 1979). This reported dissatisfaction may well be related to the many changes required in established routines and roles. When a baby is born, the parents experience a loss of free time because the child requires constant supervision. The division of labor may require a complete renegotiation. The couple must reset their patterns of interaction to include the new child, and this may bring about conflicts of interest and unexpected jealousies (Nock, 1987). The addition of a "child" position to the family system brings about role changes for the parents. All of these changes may result in surprising conflict and stress. The surprise may be especially great if the couple had idealized the prospect of becoming parents and expected it to be a purely positive experience.

For some families these changes and conflicts will be resolved readily and the transition to parenthood will be a smooth one. "Successful transitions to parenthood are based in part on the level of adjustment that couples have achieved already in their marriages" (Vincent, 1979, p. 3). In stable, adaptive relationships the partners have developed a distribution of "costs and benefits" that is reciprocal. They have developed workable patterns of roles and power distribution, and have acquired skills for changing in response to pressures. Such families are often characterized by skillful communication, good "change skills," appropriate expectations, and an infant who matches their expectations (Vincent, 1979).

Other couples may not make the transition as well. In these families, difficulty in managing change may result from an attempt to avoid conflict (Vincent, 1979). Rather than trying to negotiate a new division of labor when the new baby is taking a great deal of one partner's time, they may just try to "muddle through" until the stress becomes too great and an explosion of some sort occurs.

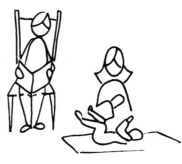

For all families who are going through this transition to parenthood the availability of outside support systems usually facilitates the transition (Vincent, 1979). If they live within a supportive community or an extended family structure, there will frequently be a role model to follow or at least someone with whom to share concerns and frustrations.

As a family deals with the transition to parenthood, child-rearing practices develop. Kagan (1984) reports that there are five mechanisms of socialization that are frequently developed as part of the parents' child-rearing practices. These mechanisms are:

1. the parents' provision of opportunities for the child to observe desirable behaviors in people in general
2. punishment of the child
3. praise of the child
4. withdrawal from the child of emotional support and signs of value
5. the parents' provision of a model with which the child can identify

Different parents adopt different mechanisms at various times. What parents teach their children using these practices depends on the culture in which the children are being raised.

FAMILY VARIATIONS

Every family deals with the issues presented earlier in this chapter. Chinese, Native American, Anglo-Saxon, single parent, extended, or traditional nuclear—every family has positions, roles, and developmental tasks. These dynamics undergird each family with whom the clinician works. Despite the similarities, there are also great differences in the kind of expectations and interventions that are appropriate in the context of each family. Some of these differences are based on cultural, socioeconomic, and family composition variations.

Stonestreet, Johnston, and Acton (1991) observe that families today are more likely to be smaller (one to two children), to represent broken homes and/or multiple marriages, and to be dysfunctional families, than in previous years. Also, American society is rapidly becoming more diverse as the percentage of nonwhite, nonAnglo citizens increases. Hanson, Lynch, and Wayman (1990) predict that "in the coming years, nearly 50 percent of all young children in many areas of the country will be from cultural and language groups that are different from those of most early intervention professionals" (p. 16). The variations in family structure and roles in different cultures are becoming an important consideration for anyone who works with families or wishes to understand them.

It is an unfortunate fact that nobody, no matter how knowledgeable or well traveled, can know all of the important characteristics of every culture encountered in work with families. Given this fact, Anderson (1991) has proposed that instead of trying to learn about every culture, clinicians can increase their general cultural sensitivity toward cultures that are different from their own. They can do this by:

1. learning what culture involves and becoming aware of their own values and expectations
2. understanding that aspects of their culture may or may not be shared by other cultures
3. respecting other cultures and their differences
4. learning about other cultures as well as their own without stereotyping or prejudging a family on the basis of ethnicity or culture
5. respecting and appreciating each family's and individual's uniqueness.

By doing this clinicians can gain "cultural (or ethnic) competence," which Hanson et al. (1990) define as "acting in a manner that is congruent with the behavior and expectations of the members of a particular culture" (p. 126).

If you were raised in the United States it may be tempting to expect everyone you encounter to have the values that are common in American society. These values underlie an approach to early intervention which is designed to help children function more independently and to have a direct impact on the child's development (Hanson et al., 1990). However, to provide culturally sensitive family-centered services, clinicians must be aware of the family's values, especially when they differ from their own and when they may be at odds with this clinical approach. It's not possible in this chapter to catalogue all of the values of various cultures; however, a few examples will illustrate differences that might be encountered.

Few sweeping generalizations can be made about individuals from any given cultural background; people are just too different. Still, commonalities can be found among people from various cultures. Western society, with contemporary American society being one of its most prominent examples, has a number of characteristics that distinguish it from other societies. Kagan (1984) reports that there are at least four ways in which Western society is distinctive. First, Western society teaches children that they, not the family, are responsible for their ". . . survival, personal reputation and material success" (p. 243). American society's respect for women is a second distinction. This attitude is related to such things as Americans' reverence for romantic love rather than arranged marriages. The ". . . celebration of freedom and selfhood of children" (p. 244) is a third distinguishing characteristic. Western society is a child-centered one in which parents are expected to sacrifice for children. Finally, ". . . Americans place greater value on sincerity and personal honesty than on social harmony . . . primary loyalty is to the self . . ." (pp. 244-245). Other societies place more value on the good of society in general than on the individual. In contemporary America, ideal qualities which parents attempt to promote in their children are often autonomy, intelligence, humaneness, sociability, and control of fear (Kagan, 1984). Although these values are seldom expressed, they may have a strong influence on parental action and attitudes in treatment situations. These values create a culture that ". . . is characterized by independence, a belief in one's own control of the environment, self-help, a change or action orientation, and a direct approach to people and issues" (Hanson et al., 1990, p. 112).

Cheng (1987) points out some of the characteristics of Asian American families. The typical Asian American family is an extended one with three or four generations closely allied. The role of each family member is clearly defined and the father is the head of the family. The mother usually stays at home with the children. Asians view the individual as part of society, with the harmony of society being more important than the individual. Communication is to be accomplished with the fewest words possible, and nonverbal cues are very important to the message. Hanson et al. (1990) report that touch is especially important in early mother-child interaction and is preferred to vocal stimulation.

Asian American families may view disability as a punishment for sins, as the result of evil spirits, or of an imbalance of "yin and yang." The family is responsible for the person with a disability and bears the guilt and shame that may be associated with the problem. Some families accept the disability as their lot in life and do not seek intervention. If intervention is considered appropriate, they may prefer to seek it within the family or ethnic community (Hanson et al., 1990).

Harrison and Alvy (1982) have similarly addressed the African American family in American society. African American or black families are generally characterized by strong kinship bonds, a strong work orientation, adaptable family roles, high achievement orientation, and strong religious ties. Family structures in the black community tend to be flexible. The majority of black families (55 percent) have both a male and female parent in the home, however 45 percent of the families have a single parent who is often the female. The most common authority pattern is the egalitarian, rather than matriarchal or patriarchal. Extended families are common in the black community; these families provide emotional, social, and material support for all members. They are usually multigenerational and headed by a dominant family figure.

African American infants are often indulged, cuddled, and played with by all members of the family. They are encouraged to be assertive and to meet their own needs. By the age of three, children are often cared for by an older sibling (Hanson et al., 1990).

Westby (1987) presents some interesting differences in caregiving patterns among various groups. In the white, middle-class, nuclear family the baby is under the primary care of the mother or father. They make all of the decisions about care and even grandparents and other close relatives frequently must ask permission to pick up the baby. In the lower socioeconomic white and black communities of the Carolinas (studied by Heath, 1983), things were done differently.

> In the White community, infants were born into the extended family. If the infant was a first child, an older woman in the family, such as a grandmother or aunt, assumed considerable care of the infant. This is, in part, a means to train the young mother in child-rearing practices and how to talk to infants. In the Black community, the infant was born into the community. Anyone in the community had the right to pick the infant up, poke it and prod it, and discipline it. (Westby, 1987, p. 9)

In the Hispanic American culture, the extended family is highly valued. The eldest male in an Hispanic American family generally holds the position of authority. Modesty and privacy are valued, but physical closeness and touching are encouraged (Food and Nutrition Service and Public Health Service, undated; Taylor, 1987). Babies tend to be kept in close physical contact and early indulgence and gratification are common. Goals for socialization include cooperativeness and harmony within the family and society rather than desire for material wealth (Hanson et al., 1990). The family is responsible for the care of elderly, young, or ill family members. As with some Asian families, Hispanics may see illness or disability as a punishment placed upon them (Food and Nutrition Service and Public Health Service, undated).

Exhibits 1-1, 1-2, and 1-3 present summaries of information from various sources related to (1) attitudes toward families, children, and childrearing tendencies, (2) tendencies in communication and interaction, and (3) attitudes and beliefs concerning health, disability, and intervention for people from Asian American, African American, and Hispanic American groups. In all cases the information in

---

Exhibit 1-1 Attitudes toward Families, Children, and Child-Rearing Tendencies

Asian Americans
- Strict gender and age hierarchy
- Father—the family leader, head of family
- Mother—the nurturer, caregiver
- Older males superior to younger males
- Females submissive to males
- Close, extended families
- Multigenerational families
- Older children strictly controlled, restricted, protected
- Physical punishment used
- Parents actively promote learning activities at home—may not participate in school functions
- Children are treasured
- Infant/toddler needs met immediately or anticipated
- Close physical contact between mother and child
- Touch rather than vocal/verbal is primary vehicle of early mother-infant interaction
- Harmony of society more important than individual
- Infant seen as independent and needing to develop dependence on family and society

African Americans
- Mothers and grandmothers may be greatest influences
- Strong extended family ties encouraged
- Independence and assertiveness encouraged
- Infants may be focus of family attention
- Affectionate treatment of babies, but fear of "spoiling"
- Strong belief in discipline, often physical
- Caregiving of older toddlers may be done by an older child

Hispanic Americans
- Strong identification with extended family
- Families tend to be patriarchal with males making most decisions
- Infants tend to be indulged; toddlers are expected to learn acceptable behavior
- Emphasis placed on cooperativeness and harmony in family and society
- Independence and ability to defend self encouraged
- Older siblings often participate in child care

Source: From *Serving Culturally Diverse Families of Infants and Toddlers with Disabilities* by P. Anderson and E. Fenichel, 1989, Washington, DC: National Center for Clinical Infant Programs; "Cultural Differences Affecting Communicative Development" by C. Westby, 1987, Rockville, MD: ASHA; "Clinical Practice as a Social Occasion" by O. Taylor, 1987, Rockville, MD: ASHA; "Honoring the Cultural Diversity of Families When Gathering Data" by M. Hanson et al., 1990, Austin, TX: PRO-ED; and *Cross-Cultural Counseling: A Guide for Nutrition and Health Counselors* by Food & Nutrition Service and Public Health Service (undated), Washington, DC: U.S. Department of Agriculture and U.S. Department of Health and Human Services.

Exhibit 1-2 Tendencies in Communication and Interaction

Asian Americans
- Communication accomplished with fewest possible words
- May drop eyes to show respect
- Direct eye contact may be considered rude
- Oldest person should be addressed first
- Casual dress may be seen as a sign of disrespect
- May agree rather than question in authority
- May be offended by use of first name only or nickname
- Paternal grandmother may play a decision-making role

African Americans
- May be little vocalization to infant
- Infants may be expected to learn language by observation
- May prefer physical touching and closeness within the cultural group
- May avert eyes during listening; use direct eye contact when speaking

Hispanic Americans
- May use close proximity and frequent touching during conversation
- Mothers may use a relatively high degree of vocalization with infants
- Older siblings may provide much of the language input for toddlers
- Conversational patterns may be taught using modeled messages to be repeated to a third person, e.g., "Tell him, 'I want juice' "
- Infants expected to learn language by observation, not seen as having intentional control over early language behavior

Source: From *Serving Culturally Diverse Families of Infants and Toddlers with Disabilities* by P. Anderson and E. Fenichel, 1989, Washington, DC: National Center for Clinical Infant Programs; "Cultural Differences Affecting Communicative Development" by C. Westby, 1987, Rockville, MD: ASHA; "Clinical Practice as a Social Occasion" by O. Taylor, 1987, Rockville, MD: ASHA; "Honoring the Cultural Diversity of Families When Gathering Data" by M. Hanson et al., 1990, Austin, TX: PRO-ED; and *Cross-Cultural Counseling: A Guide for Nutrition and Health Counselors* by Food & Nutrition Service and Public Health Service (undated), Washington, DC: U.S. Department of Agriculture and U.S. Department of Health and Human Services.

Exhibits 1-1, 1-2, and 1-3 should be considered to represent general tendencies of groups of people rather than behaviors to be expected from specific clients.

If early intervention practitioners are unaware of some of these cultural differences, they may misinterpret communications or other behaviors. A vivid illustration of this danger is given by Hanson et al. (1990).

One example of a traditional practice that has led to misunderstandings in the American culture is the use of coin rubbing. This massage treatment is utilized by the Vietnamese community to treat disorders

Exhibit 1-3 Attitudes and Beliefs Concerning Health, Disability, and Intervention

Asian Americans
- Disabilities may be viewed as punishment for sins of the parents or ancestors or as the result of evil spirits or an imbalance of *yin and yang*
- Family may be ashamed and isolate the child with a disability
- May take a fatalistic attitude
- May not seek or accept intervention or only seek help within the family or ethnic community
- Privacy and respectful treatment are very important in interactions

African Americans
(Little information available)
- May have experienced problems with health care and long waits for services
- May believe in the "evil eye" as a cause of harm

Hispanic Americans
- Health and vitality are highly prized
- Infants with disabilities may be hidden or indulged by family
- Illness may be seen as result of imbalance in physical and social factors
- Mind and body seen as linked
- Illness or disability may be seen as punishment of a parent's wrongs or as the work of evil forces
- Families accept responsibility of care for elderly, young, or ill family members

Source: From *Serving Culturally Diverse Families of Infants and Toddlers with Disabilities* by P. Anderson and E. Fenichel, 1989, Washington, DC: National Center for Clinical Infant Programs; "Cultural Differences Affecting Communicative Development" by C. Westby, 1987, Rockville, MD: ASHA; "Clinical Practice as a Social Occasion" by O. Taylor, 1987, Rockville, MD: ASHA; "Honoring the Cultural Diversity of Families When Gathering Data" by M. Hanson et al., 1990, Austin, TX: PRO-ED; and *Cross-Cultural Counseling: A Guide for Nutrition and Health Counselors* by Food & Nutrition Service and Public Health Service (undated), Washington, DC: U.S. Department of Agriculture and U.S. Department of Health and Human Services.

such as headaches and colds. Coin treatment, or Cao Gio, literally translates to scratching the (bad) wind out of the body. The treatment involves the massaging of chest and back with a medicated substance, like Ben-Gay, and the striking or scratching of the skin with a coin or spoon. This process leaves superficial bruises and, when spotted by professionals who are unaware of the technique, has often resulted in a referral for child abuse. This practice provides a clear example of differences in treatment techniques used by Western medicine and other cultures and also dramatically underscores the issues in diagnosis and interpretation when the various cultures meet. (p. 122)

An awareness of our own cultural values and practices and those of the families with which we work will help to prevent misunderstanding and to promote quality care for children.

Within any of these or other cultural or socioeconomic settings there may also be variations in family composition. Even in societies that value the traditional nuclear family or the extended family, variations occur. Single parent and blended families (made up of parents and children who are not all biologically related) are becoming increasingly common. Each variation may have its own added difficulties in role definitions for family members and complication of developmental task mastery.

These examples make it clear that there are many different family structures and expectations that play important roles in the developmental contexts of infants and young children.

THE FAMILY AS A SYSTEM

The idea that a family functions as a system has been explored in several of the previous sections of this chapter. The concepts of nurturing versus troubled and functional versus dysfunctional family systems were discussed, as was the idea of the family system being balanced much like a mobile. There are still a number of aspects of the family system that have not yet been explored. Satir's (1972) conception of the family system is an especially helpful one.

> Any system consists of several individual parts that are essential and related to one another when a certain outcome is desired. There are actions and reactions and interactions among the parts that keep changing. Each part acts as a starter to all the other parts. It is this constant action, reaction, and interaction that form the most important part of my concept of system. A system has life only *now* when the component parts are there to give it. (p. 112)

The family system has a purpose or goal (protecting and socializing the members), parts (the mother, father, children), an orderly plan for the working of the parts (communication, child-rearing practices, rules), a way of starting the system (conception of the first child), power or energy to keep the parts working (food, shelter), and ways of dealing with changes (interacting with and adjusting to the new and different) (Satir, 1972).

While all family systems have these common elements, they may also be quite different. Satir (1972, 1988) sees families as being either closed or open systems. Closed systems are rigid; they are based on power and rules and performance is all-important. Open systems are much more flexible and self-worth is of primary importance.

In addition to the total family system with all of its separate human units, the structure of the family also has subsystems of people who interact with each other. There are four major subsystems in the traditional family system: (1) the marital (husband-wife); (2) the parental (parent-child); (3) the sibling (child-child); and (4) the extrafamilial (family member(s)-nonfamily member(s)) subsystem(s) (Turnbull and Turnbull, 1986). Other subsystems may also develop; for example, two parental subsystems, one of Mom and an at-risk infant, and another of Dad and two older, normally developing children, might develop in a family which is participating in early intervention.

Both the family system and each of the subsystems in a family may be seen as having a certain degree of cohesion. Cohesion is ". . . the emotional bonding that members have toward each other and the independence of an individual within the family system" (Turnbull and Turnbull, 1986, p. 61). This cohesion can be viewed as varying from extreme disengagement (each unit acting separately) to extreme enmeshment (units interacting constantly).

The family system and each of its subsystems also have their own interpersonal boundaries which regulate the amount of contact that the system or subsystem has with others. Boundaries are important in that they safeguard the autonomy of the system by regulating the amount of contact between the system and outside influences (Nichols, 1988).

The system boundaries may be rigid or diffuse, or fall anywhere on a continuum from one extreme to the other (Minuchin, 1974). When a boundary is rigid it permits little contact with other systems, subsystems, or individuals. This rigidity results in disengagement, with disengaged systems or subsystems being independent and isolated from one another (Nichols, 1988; Turnbull and Turnbull, 1986). For example, in the Mom-infant and Dad-older siblings subsystems mentioned earlier, if the Mom-infant subsystem becomes involved in its own interaction, leaving little time or energy to interact with Dad and the older children, rigid boundaries may develop between the two subsystems. These boundaries may make interaction between the subsystems difficult even when Mom is not interacting with the infant. On the positive side, disengagement fosters development of individual skills and personal self-reliance, but on the negative side, it makes warmth and nurturance more difficult (Nichols, 1988).

If systems or subsystems have diffuse boundaries, there is little protection from outside influences and a great deal of interaction between systems and subsystems. When system boundaries are diffuse or weak, family members may become enmeshed; that is, they may experience a great deal of support and involvement with one another, but little privacy, autonomy, or independence (Nichols, 1988; Turnbull and Turnbull, 1986).

This kind of interaction feels warm and loving, but family members may become overinvolved in each others' lives, parents may be overprotective, and it may be difficult for children to develop a sense of self or to feel comfortable by themselves at an appropriate age (Nichols, 1988; Turnbull and Turnbull, 1986). For example, if the Dad-older children subsystem of the family we have been discussing (which is actually made up of three subsystems—Dad and child number 1, Dad and child number 2, and child number 1 and child number 2) becomes enmeshed, each of the three smaller subsystems will have diffuse boundaries. The result may be a great deal of three-way interaction but little privacy or permission for the children to "just be kids" together; Dad may always feel compelled to help them settle arguments or to make all activities family centered. Another outcome of this enmeshed interaction may be that the Mom and the at-risk infant may be shut out of the family activities, leading to greater family system imbalance.

Family systems can also be considered adaptable or rigid in this response to forces that lead to change. Rigid families are highly controlled and structured and resistant to change. Some families change so readily that they are unstable or chaotic. These families have little control or structure and family members may not be able to depend on one another (Turnbull and Turnbull, 1986).

Turnbull and Turnbull (1986) organize the components of the family system into input, process, and output. The inputs to the system are the family resources, its characteristics, size, culture, socioeconomic status, location, etc. The process of the system is family interaction which can be viewed in terms of its cohesion and adaptability. The outputs of the family are its functions, e.g., economic support, recreation, socialization, etc. Influencing these components is the family life cycle with its changes and stresses including any characteristics of exceptionality (e.g., developmental delay, illness) of any of the family members.

For a complete, contextual view of the family and any of its members, it may be helpful also to consider Bronfenbrenner's (1977) idea of an ecological environment. Bronfenbrenner views each person as developing in relationship to changing environments. These ecological environments are systems that relate to other systems. The microsystem is the family as we have been discussing it, the individual's immediate setting. The mesosystem includes the relationships among the individual's major settings: home, school, and peer group. The exosystem is made up of other social structures that impinge on the individual's environments, such as the mass media, government, and the like. The highest level of all of these influential systems is the macrosystem. The macrosystem is made up of the general prototypes (laws, ideologies) of the culture that set the pattern for activities and life events (Bronfenbrenner, 1977). When an individual is viewed within the family system and within these larger systems, we gain a more complete picture of the important influences on development.

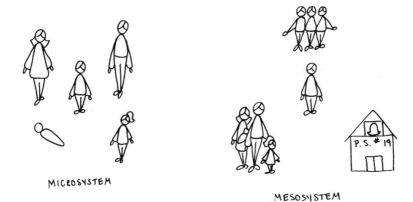

MICROSYSTEM

MESOSYSTEM

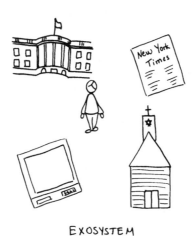

EXOSYSTEM

CONCLUSION

This chapter examined several aspects of the family system, its nature, function, development, and variations. The next chapter will look at the family's role as a context for communication development. It will discuss the characteristics of family life in light of the child's requirements for optimal language learning.

2

The Family As a Context for Communication Development

One of the functions of the family system which was discussed in the previous chapter is to socialize children, to introduce them to the culture in which they are to live so that they understand the expectations of that culture and can operate by its rules. One aspect of any human culture is its language. Clinicians who are especially interested in communication and its development may think of the parents, or more broadly, the family, as having the specific purpose of helping their child to learn language and communication skills. What they more likely are trying to do is to make their child "civilized" in the eyes of their community. What is really being learned is a code for interacting with and within their specific culture.

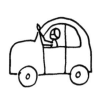 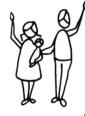 Bruner (1983) points out that we master language so that we can interpret and regulate the culture. "Children begin to use language . . . not because they have a language-using capacity, but because they need to get things done by its use. Parents assist them in a like spirit: they want to help them become 'civilized' human beings, not just speakers of the language" (p. 104). But how does the family accomplish this aspect of socialization? What is there about the family environment and the infant's interaction with that environment that helps a child to learn language?

WHAT ROLE THE ENVIRONMENT PLAYS— THE MAJOR THEORIES

During the past two decades, many significantly different theories of how a child acquires language have been proposed. One interesting thread of difference between the theories that can be followed is that of the importance ascribed to various aspects of the child's environment during language learning.

The oldest theory of language acquisition is the one first propounded by St. Augustine and later embellished by behaviorists such as B.F. Skinner (Bruner, 1983). In this theory, the child's environment plays an all-important role in language acquisition. To oversimplify, adults (or older children) in the child's environment present stimuli (e.g., objects paired with words) to the child who responds by imitating the words and is then reinforced by the adult. The environment here is of prime importance—no language could be acquired without active participation of the adult or older child who models and reinforces language behavior.

In contrast to the behaviorist point of view, psycholinguists, such as Noam Chomsky who emphasized the importance of language structure, minimize the importance of environmental influences on language acquisition. These theorists hypothesize that an innate, language-specific learning capacity called the "language acquisition device" (LAD), which is assumed to be part of the child's brain, allows the child to learn language even if there is little input from the environment (Chomsky, 1965). No special models or responses from adults are considered necessary in this theory; the environment plays a minor role in language development.

The cognitive-interactionist (psycholinguistic semantic/cognitive) theory of language acquisition views the environment as an important contributor to language acquisition, because the child gains the cognitive prerequisites for language use through sensory-motor interaction with the environment. Specific linguistic inputs or adjustments of the language model are not necessary as long as the environment promotes development of the cognitive structures that underlie language as one form of symbolic behavior.

Perhaps the most inclusive and currently popular theory of language learning is the social interactionist approach. This approach gives nearly equal importance to the child as an "active and specialized language processor" (Bohannon and Warren-Leubecker, 1989, p. 187) and to the environment as a provider of experience and linguistic input and response. In addition, this view appreciates the bidirectional influences on communicative interactions, recognizing that while the caregivers provide specific language input and response for the child, certain characteristics of the child influence the kind of input and response that the caregivers provide. This viewpoint further emphasizes the social role of language and the role that social interaction plays in promoting language growth. Language is viewed as having an important structure, as in other theories, but the functions of language are given even greater emphasis. The ability to use language in social interaction is considered a prime motivator for its acquisition.

Bruner (1983) suggested some interesting aspects of this social interactionist theme. Bruner accepted the necessity of a "predisposing set of language-learning capacities" (p. 19) such as Chomsky's LAD, but disagreed that the

LAD can operate almost independent of special environmental inputs and responses. The child, in Bruner's theory, needs an adult who will provide a "language acquisition support system" (LASS) that demonstrates and responds to the use of language: ". . . it is the interaction between LAD and LASS that makes it possible for the infant to enter the linguistic community . . ." (p. 19). Adults don't just model language for the child, they "negotiate" with the child about the form of his or her communication and the conditions under which it may be used. They impose "felicity conditions" that dictate their culture's rules for communication. The adult's role is to help to make the child's intentions clear and to make his or her speech fit the requirements of the culture.

This review of the hypothesized importance of the environment to language learning in the various theories is not a comprehensive overview of each theory. For a more complete examination of the theories, refer to Bohannon and Warren-Leubecker (1989) or Rice (1989).

Clearly, the preponderance of theories argue for the importance of certain aspects of the child's environment to language learning. In the next section of the chapter we will consider what aspects of family life may facilitate language acquisition and development.

THE FAMILY AS A MEDIUM FOR COMMUNICATION GROWTH

The social interactionist view of the importance of both what the child brings to the language learning experience and what the environment provides as a context presents a useful construct for further consideration of the family. The family "people-making" system creates a multifaceted environment in which a child is nurtured and grows. The family provides a growth medium or "soil" for cultivating the child's communication abilities. What is there about the family environment that makes it an especially good place to "grow" communication skills?

The family can be seen as providing four forms of input to the communication learning process. The first can be thought of as stimuli for developmental interaction. These stimuli consist of the world of people, things, and events that the child learns about in the process of cognitive and social development. The second is the need and desire to communicate. The family provides conditions that stimulate the child's need to use various forms of communication, as well as the desire to communicate with family members. A third form of input, communication/language models and opportunities, consists of family members' communication and language behavior that can be imitated or otherwise used as data for the language-learning system, as well as chances to use language and other forms of communication in a familiar context. The fourth form of input from the family is *consequences* for attempts at communication.

These are responses to, or other sequelae of, the child's communication behaviors. These components are displayed in Table 2-1.

All of these inputs take place within and are influenced by the family system and the physical and greater social environment within which that family system exists. Consideration of each of these inputs may help us to identify essential characteristics of the family as a language-learning context, as will be discussed later.

Stimuli for Developmental Interaction

Every family, regardless of culture, socioeconomic status (SES), or constitution, creates a world of people, things, and events within which its members live and develop. For the child who is in the process of learning to communicate, these become the context within which he or she learns about the world. In interaction with the objects and people in the environment, children master the cognitive correlates of language. The 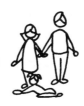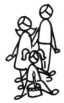 physical terrain of the environment provides the context for motor development. The family members, especially the primary caregiver, engage in interac-

Table 2-1 Contributions of the Family Environment to Language Learning

Component of the Environment	Benefit to the Child
Stimuli for developmental interaction	Expose the child to people, things, and events which stimulate cognitive and social development
Conditions that produce need and desire to communicate	Stimulate use of the various functions of communication
Communication/language models and opportunities	Can be imitated or used as a chance to practice communication skills
Consequences of communication attempts	Serve to reinforce or punish and therefore increase or modify behavior

tions with the child that allow him or her to learn about self and others, and to develop expectations for general social relations. Events, both daily routines and the extraordinary happenings of holidays, family celebrations, trips, or vacations, present the child with information about the workings of the social and physical world. All of these stimuli are part of the family context. They allow the child to learn about the world in general and his or her role in his or her own world in particular. This world knowledge provides, among other things, the basis for the semantic aspect of language development—the basis for meaning.

EXERCISE #1

Think for a few moments about the stimuli available to a child in your family or in some other family that you know well. Now consider a family whose income is below the poverty level, perhaps a family who lives in the most economically depressed section of your town. How would the stimuli available to a young child in that family differ from those available in the first family you considered? How might the differences affect language learning in the two families?

Conditions That Produce Need and Desire To Communicate

A second important aspect of the family context is the motivation it provides for the use of communication. As the infant's earliest attempts at reducing tension by squirming, crying, and smiling are interpreted as meaningful communicative acts, he or she begins to understand the power of these behaviors and to use them intentionally.

To gain some insight into the family's role in this process we must look closely at the infant's early days and months as a member of that family. The human neonate is, of course, incapable of self-defense or self-care. Even self-regulation is a difficult task. It is imperative that the vulnerable infant be cared for by someone older and more capable. Because the neonate cannot cling to or follow its caregiver, it must have some means of keeping that caregiver close and interested in giving care. Signals such as crying and smiling, in addition to the appeal of its physically helpless appearance, have become important promoters of the necessary proximity (Kaplan, 1978; Lamb, Thompson, Gardner, Charnov, & Connell, 1985). When these primitive means of communication meet with success, the infant is afforded the opportunity to develop even more sophisticated ways of conveying his or her needs.

The infant-primary caregiver dyad, which is held together by mutual attachment (to be discussed later), develops a complicated, largely nonverbal system of communication called a "dialogue" (Greenspan & Greenspan, 1985; Kaplan, 1978; Spitz, 1965). In the context of this dialogue each member of the dyad learns how best to stimulate and respond to the other partner—which tone of voice and movement brings a smile, what body posture or gesture will prolong interest and interaction. It is a dialogue of action and response rather than words, with the older partner often acting as interpreter for the infant. As Kaplan (1978) stated

> When the baby enters the new world, he has a language—the inborn gestures and potentials that give him a readiness to reach out, to discover the world, and eventually to create his own knowledge about the world. But he needs an interpreter who can make what he is ready to receive sensible and real. (p. 87)

In addition to interpreting the world for the infant, the caregiver interprets the infant's communications to the world. Long before the child intends to tell of his dislike of some substance or texture by grimacing, the caregiver interprets and verbalizes this communication for the child (e.g., "Oh, this is different cereal today isn't it? You don't like it as much as rice cereal, do you? This is funny tasting stuff."). By being treated as a communicator, the child learns how to communicate (Greenfield, 1969). His or her various needs are recognized, talked about, and often met by the caregiver, demonstrating ways of making a whole range of intentions clear. Requests, greetings, and declarations all have ways of being expressed and understood.

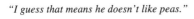

"I guess that means he doesn't like peas."

In a responsive environment, a child's innate ability to communicate by nonverbal means is eventually transformed into the ability to communicate verbally. The needs communicated and the need to communicate are both met through interaction with various family members. The desire to communicate seems to grow out of these need-meeting situations, but it continues long after the caregivers have ceased to be necessary for the child's survival. Desire to communicate seems to be closely related to the development of the child's relationship to the primary caregiver(s), which includes the phenomenon of attachment and the process through which the child develops a sense of self as separate from others. These ideas will be discussed later in this chapter.

EXERCISE #2

Again, imagine children learning language in two different family situations. Imagine first a family that Satir might describe as "nurturing" or which we might call "functional" (see Chapter 1 for a review of these concepts). Then consider a family in which there is a particularly high level of stress created by some situation—enough stress to make the family "troubled" or "dysfunctional." How might the infant's experience in regard to need and desire to communicate differ in these two families? How could that affect language learning?

Communication/Language Models and Opportunities

A great deal of attention has been given to the role of the language model in child language acquisition. There is little doubt that having clearly and frequently presented demonstrations of how to communicate according to the rules of the culture is essential to learning this complex process. It is also clear that a family context can be a very good setting for exposure to such a model. Because transactions in the family system require both nonverbal and verbal communication, children both participate in and observe communicative interaction.

Research has shown that much of the speech addressed to language-learning children, at least in Western society, comes in a form that is somewhat different from adult-adult discourse. This specially tailored, child-directed language, or "motherese" (Newport, 1976), appears to be adapted so that it exposes the child to the characteristics of the language. Motherese, which is spoken not just by mothers but by most people (as young as four) who address children in the language-learning process, has several reliable characteristics: (1) pitch is raised and exaggerated, (2) pauses occur between utterances, (3) sentences are shorter, simpler, and more fluent, (4) vocabulary is more concrete and redundant, (5) utterances are repeated and paraphrased, (6) the child's utterances are often expanded (repeated in a more grammatically complete form), (7) utterances are based on the same semantic relations that children of this age use, (8) there are more questions and fewer comments than in adult-adult speech, and (9) topics usually pertain to the "here and now" and are often contingent upon (on the same topic as) the child's activities or previous utterances (Chapman, 1982). These adjustments also appear to depend upon the child's specific level of understanding and production of the language rather than occurring simply as a general response to small children or deficient language users (Chapman, 1982).

Motherese seems to be one aspect of what Bruner (1983) calls the "language acquisition support system" (LASS). But, as Bruner points out, this support system is more than just a nicely adapted model of language. The adult interacts with the child and constructs situations which give the child the opportunity to experience being a language user. Bruner (1983) defines four aspects of the LASS.

First, the adult highlights interesting features of the world that have basic or simple grammatical form. These are often presented in formats built around games or other routines.

Second, the adult encourages and models lexical and phrase substitutes for gestures and vocalizations. The child develops a number of "scripts," complete with directions for "communicative procedures" to use in them (p. 41).

Third, the play formats later become "pretend" situations; they are good opportunities for language learning and practice.

Fourth, the routinized formats generalize from one situation (or even one communicative intention) to another.

Throughout the communicative interactions the child is an active participant who influences the adult's verbal and nonverbal communication and who communicates in response, at first nonverbally, then on both verbal and nonverbal levels.

EXERCISE #3

- Think for a few minutes about cultural differences in the communication/language models furnished for the language-learning child. (For further information on this topic see Lieven [1984] or Schieffelin & Eisenberg [1984].)

- How might the language models and communication opportunities be different in families where the mother is the primary caregiver for a toddler and in families where older siblings may provide much of a toddler's care as is the case in some of the cultures discussed in Chapter 1?

- What effect might this have on language learning?

Consequences of Communication Attempts

As important as appropriate levels of stimulation and a specially adapted language model are to the language-learning process, the responses that family members give to the child's attempts at communication are at least as important. When the child attempts to communicate, people in the environment can 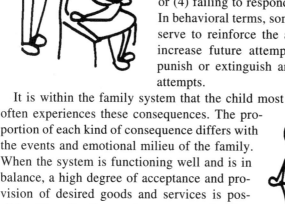 respond or they can fail to respond. All of the behaviors that follow the child's communication attempts can act as consequences of that attempt. Possible consequences that family members may provide include: (1) accepting (providing a positive response to) or rejecting (providing a negative response to) the attempt; (2) interrupting it; (3) providing desired goods or services to the child; or (4) failing to respond in any discernible way. In behavioral terms, some of these consequences serve to reinforce the attempt and therefore to increase future attempts, and others serve to punish or extinguish and therefore to decrease attempts.

It is within the family system that the child most often experiences these consequences. The proportion of each kind of consequence differs with the events and emotional milieu of the family. When the system is functioning well and is in balance, a high degree of acceptance and provision of desired goods and services is possible. When family members are experiencing stress related to developmental tasks or role changes such as those described in Chapter 1, it may be more difficult for them to respond to attempts at communication with positive consequences. A higher rate of rejection or interruption or failures to respond may result.

All of these varieties of responses, both positive and negative, occur in any family. The regularity with which they occur is probably the significant factor for language learning. A child who regularly experiences a high proportion of accepting, satisfying consequences in response to communication attempts probably develops a greater desire to continue communicating and is likely to feel comfortable trying more difficult or demanding forms of communication in the future.

EXERCISE #4

There appear to be some different cultural tendencies in responses to children's attempts at communication. For example, cultures that promote and depend upon verbal interaction (such as Western culture) may more readily reinforce children's verbal output than cultures in which communication is to be accomplished in the fewest possible words (e.g., Asian American). Are you aware of any such differences? Discuss this with classmates, friends, or acquaintances from other cultures.

Individual families may provide more or less fertile ground for producing children who are communicatively competent. Families may differ greatly in their ability to provide the stimuli, need and desire, models, and consequences discussed above. Some of the influences that may determine a family's ability to provide fertile ground for language development will be discussed in the next section of this chapter.

SOME FACTORS THAT INFLUENCE THE FAMILY AS A GROWTH MEDIUM

The family system is clearly a complex one with many factors that are important to the development of communication skills. Several ideas which were introduced earlier appear to be especially influential in this process and will be discussed in greater detail in this section of the chapter.

All of the ideas about the family as a language-learning context would be simpler if we considered only the family's effect on the child. Unfortunately, that would sacrifice understanding and accuracy for simplicity. The child is an important influence on the family and plays an active role in all of its interactions (transactions) with him or her from the beginning.

A "transactional model" of the relationship between the child and his or her environment has been developed by Sameroff (1975, 1982). In this model, development is viewed as the result of ". . . a continual interplay between a changing organism and a changing environment" (Sameroff, 1982, p. 143). The child's characteristics and behaviors at one point in time cause a certain response in the caregiver and other aspects of the environment. The caregiving environment may in turn cause the child to respond in a slightly different way, producing a change in the child. As these transactions continue, both the child and his or her environment adapt and develop. For example, a blind infant does not give the eye contact that parents expect from an infant. This characteristic of the infant may cause the caregiver (parents) to feel rejected and consequently to respond in a more reserved or less loving manner. This reaction of the caregivers is translated into their nonverbal behavior with the child and may, in turn, cause the child to use other nonverbal behaviors (e.g., responses to tactile input such as molding to the caregiver's body when held) less successfully.

The nature and process of these early transactions between the infant and the caregivers seem especially important to our understanding of the development of the child's communication abilities within the family context. Through these continually adjusted transactions the child and caregivers develop their relationship. McLean (1990) views early communication development as a result of this transactional process. In this model of development the

> . . . infant's observable responses are seen to serve as both the antecedent events that evoke subsequent responses from the environment; and as the consequent events that either reinforce or punish (i.e., increase or decrease the rate of) those subsequent environmental events. Similarly, environmental events, consisting primarily of caregiver responses, also serve dual functions as both antecedent and consequent events, evoking and rewarding (or punishing) the infant's responses. (p. 14)

With these mutually adjusted antecedent and consequent events, the infant and caregiver influence each other's developing communication behaviors. In this way the infant develops three related sets of communication behaviors: production skills, comprehension skills, and dyadic/discourse skills. Production skills include the expressive behaviors available to the infant during different stages of development, including nonverbal behaviors such as crying, smiling, and vocalizing, as well as expressive language and speech skills. Comprehension skills are those skills that allow the infant to derive meaning from symbolic forms such as speech and nonsymbolic nonverbal behaviors (e.g., smiling, touching, and tone of voice). Dyadic/discourse skills include abilities such as turn taking, topic control, presupposition, and the use of polite forms of address.

McLean (1990) traces these three components of communication through four stages of development using the transactional model as a framework (Exhibit 2-1). At each of these stages the child is capable of a certain level of production, comprehension, and discourse. Stage I, which extends from birth to two or three months, is the stage of Reactive Perlocutionary Communication. This stage is characterized by the infant's reflexive reactions to internal and external stimuli. The caregiver responds by assigning meaning to these responses and adjusting the level of input to suit the infant. The most important aspect of the caregiver's verbal communication to the infant is its intonation or paralinguistic features. The term *perlocutionary* signifies that the infant's behaviors are not yet intentional communication behaviors but they are interpreted as communicative by the caregiver.

In Stage II, which extends from two to three months to eight to nine months, infants engage in Proactive Perlocutionary Communication. The infant's nonverbal behaviors (e.g., reaching, grasping, vocalizing) of this stage are more purposeful and volitionally controlled. The behaviors are still not used intentionally as communicative behaviors, however, and are still interpreted by the caregiver. The caregiver begins to put more stress on the words he or she uses with the infant, usually talking about what the infant is attending to.

Stage III, the stage of Emerging Illocutionary Communication, lasts from eight or nine months to 12 to 15 months. This stage marks the beginning of intentional communication on the part of the infant, and is therefore labeled *illocutionary*. This intentional communication is characterized by coordinated attention to the caregiver and to the thing the infant wants to have done or attended to (e.g., reaching toward a desired object while looking at the caregiver and vocalizing). The caregiver now "fine tunes" his or her language input to the child's level of comprehension and models the appropriate linguistic forms for the child's apparent intentions.

In Stage IV, Conventional Illocutionary and Emerging Locutionary Communication, which extends from 12 to 15 months through 18 to 24 months, the toddler uses conventional gestures and intonations as well as proto-words (consistently used sound patterns) and words to communicate on an increasingly linguistic or *locutionary* level. The caregiver continues to adapt his or her input to the toddler's needs with semantically contingent speech that follows the toddler's attention and expands his or her utterances.

The general process of early interaction has been studied by many researchers and from many different points of view. Observational and experimental studies of parent-child interaction (usually mother-child interaction) have been done by psychoanalysts, ethologists, and learning theorists, as well as researchers who appear to take an eclectic point of view which draws ideas and methodologies from all of these schools of thought.

Two very useful ideas, attachment/bonding and separation/individuation, have come from interaction research. Both of these ideas relate to the child's development of relationships with other people. The first idea, attachment/bonding, involves the process by which the child becomes psychologically tied to one or more other people and the way those people (usually parents) forge the same kind of tie to the child. It is a process of mutual "falling in love" (Greenspan & Greenspan, 1985) which is essential for healthy psychological development and even for physical well-being (Bowlby, 1969; Klaus & Kennell, 1983; Spitz, 1965).

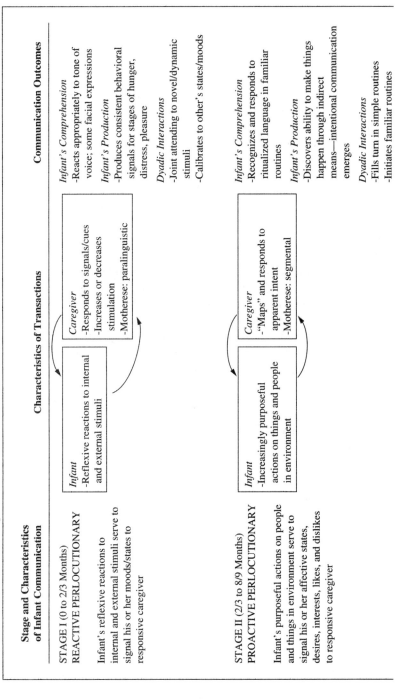

Exhibit 2-1 Communication Development from Birth to Two: A Transactional Process

Stage and Characteristics of Infant Communication	Characteristics of Transactions	Communication Outcomes
STAGE I (0 to 2/3 Months) REACTIVE PERLOCUTIONARY Infant's reflexive reactions to internal and external stimuli serve to signal his or her moods/states to responsive caregiver	*Infant* -Reflexive reactions to internal and external stimuli *Caregiver* -Responds to signals/cues -Increases or decreases stimulation -Motherese: paralinguistic	*Infant's Comprehension* -Reacts appropriately to tone of voice; some facial expressions *Infant's Production* -Produces consistent behavioral signals for stages of hunger, distress, pleasure *Dyadic Interactions* -Joint attending to novel/dynamic stimuli -Calibrates to other's states/moods
STAGE II (2/3 to 8/9 Months) PROACTIVE PERLOCUTIONARY Infant's purposeful actions on people and things in environment serve to signal his or her affective states, desires, interests, likes, and dislikes to responsive caregiver	*Infant* -Increasingly purposeful actions on things and people in environment *Caregiver* -"Maps" and responds to apparent intent -Motherese: segmental	*Infant's Comprehension* -Recognizes and responds to ritualized language in familiar routines *Infant's Production* -Discovers ability to make things happen through indirect means—intentional communication emerges *Dyadic Interactions* -Fills turn in simple routines -Initiates familiar routines

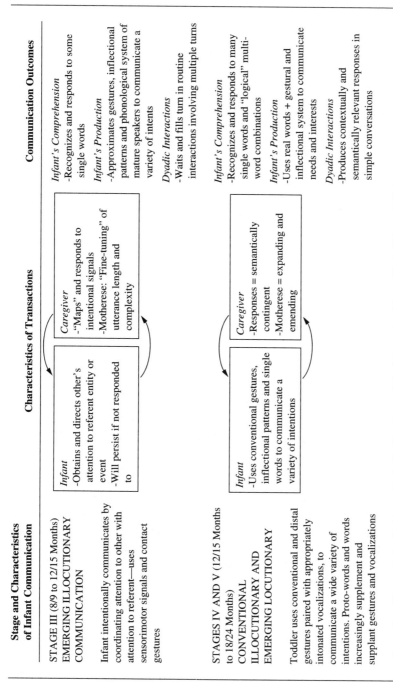

Stage and Characteristics of Infant Communication	Characteristics of Transactions	Communication Outcomes
STAGE III (8/9 to 12/15 Months) EMERGING ILLOCUTIONARY COMMUNICATION Infant intentionally communicates by coordinating attention to other with attention to referent—uses sensorimotor signals and contact gestures	*Infant* -Obtains and directs other's attention to referent entity or event -Will persist if not responded to *Caregiver* -"Maps" and responds to intentional signals -Motherese: "Fine-tuning" of utterance length and complexity	*Infant's Comprehension* -Recognizes and responds to some single words *Infant's Production* -Approximates gestures, inflectional patterns and phonological system of mature speakers to communicate a variety of intents *Dyadic Interactions* -Waits and fills turn in routine interactions involving multiple turns
STAGES IV AND V (12/15 Months to 18/24 Months) CONVENTIONAL ILLOCUTIONARY AND EMERGING LOCUTIONARY Toddler uses conventional and distal gestures paired with appropriately intonated vocalizations, to communicate a wide variety of intentions. Proto-words and words increasingly supplement and supplant gestures and vocalizations	*Infant* -Uses conventional gestures, inflectional patterns and single words to communicate a variety of intentions *Caregiver* -Responses = semantically contingent -Motherese = expanding and emending	*Infant's Comprehension* -Recognizes and responds to many single words and "logical" multi-word combinations *Infant's Production* -Uses real words + gestural and inflectional system to communicate needs and interests *Dyadic Interactions* -Produces contextually and semantically relevant responses in simple conversations

Source: From "Communication Development in the First Two Years of Life: A Transactional Process" by L. McLean, 1990, *Zero to Three, 11,* p. 15. Copyright 1990 by National Center for Clinical Infant Programs. Reprinted with permission.

Attachment/Bonding

The developing tie between child and parent can, of course, be viewed from two different sides of the process. We can concentrate on the child's growing love for the parent, or on the parent's developing affection for the child. The term *attachment* has generally been used to refer to the former, and *bonding* to the latter.

While the phenomena of attachment and bonding are certainly not new, the consideration of their importance and the scientific investigation of their development is relatively new. Until the 1930s, early experience was thought to be unimportant to later development (Lamb et al., 1985). With the psychoanalytic theories of Freud and the studies by Bowlby (1965) and Spitz (1945) of children who failed to grow and develop when they were placed in orphanages and sanatoria without a primary caregiver, these ideas began to change.

The first attempts to explain attachment grew from psychoanalytical thinkers' "secondary drive theory." This theory hypothesized that the child's feelings for mother grew from the primary drive for food; because of mother's association with food, the child develops a secondary drive for her. This idea was first brought into serious question by Harlow's studies with Rhesus monkeys in which he demonstrated that "contact comfort" was more important than food as an evoker of clinging or attachment behavior (Lamb et al., 1985).

Based on these pieces of evidence, Bowlby began to develop a theory of the development of attachment in infants. Bowlby's theory holds that infants have an innate need for social interaction that eventually becomes centered on one person (Lamb et al., 1985). Bowlby focused on child behaviors such as sucking, clinging, following, smiling, and crying, which function to maintain proximity to the mother or other "attachment figure." "Infants become attached to individuals who consistently and appropriately respond to the infant's proximity-promoting signals and behaviors" (Lamb et al., 1985, p. 13).

The child's development of a stable attachment to one or more people may be of major importance to the growth of communication ability. Not only does attachment keep the child and adult in close proximity where the dialogue can proceed and language modeling and practice can take place, attachment also seems to have a general positive effect on the infant's organization and self-regulation. "The various ways in which an infant organizes his behaviors toward his attachment figure constitute a starting point for the way in which he later organizes his behavior toward a whole series of age-appropriate developmental tasks . . ." (Ainsworth, 1985, p. 28). In addition, the child's identification with the attachment figure seems to increase the child's desire to be like that person, to stir with a spoon in a cup just like Daddy, or to use words just like Mommy. Kagan (1984) states, "I believe that the major consequence of an attachment is to make the child receptive to the adoption of parental standards because the child is reluctant to tolerate the uncertainty implied by anticipated signs of parental indifference or rejection" (p. 63).

Bowlby and his followers were primarily concerned with the child's development of a tie to the parents. The other side of the attachment issue is the parents' developing love for the child. It is tempting to assume that parents automatically love or are attached to their children as soon as they are born. Unfortunately, many parents don't feel instant love for their infants (Klaus & Kennell, 1983). Even for parents, becoming attached is a developmental process which is influenced by many factors. For some parents attachment to the child appears to begin during pregnancy (Verny & Kelly, 1981), while for others feelings of this sort do not emerge until the first week of life or even later. MacFarlane, Smith, and Garrow (1978) studied mothers' first reports of feelings of love for the baby; 41% reported love feelings during pregnancy, 24% at birth, 27% during the first week, and 8% reported that they didn't feel love until after the first week.

These differences in reaction to the child are apparently influenced by many factors which may occur before pregnancy, during pregnancy, during birth, or after birth (Klaus & Kennell, 1983). "A mother or father's behavior toward an infant is the result of a complex combination of their own genetic endowments, the infant's responses to them, a long history of interpersonal relations with their own families and with each other, past experiences with this or previous pregnancies, the absorption of the practices and values of their cultures, and probably most important of all, the way in which each was raised by his or her own parents" (Klaus & Kennell, 1983, pp. 38-39). In addition to these historical influences, Klaus and Kennell (1983) have hypothesized that events surrounding the birth may facilitate or interfere with bonding. They believe that care practices during labor and delivery can influence bonding. For example, physicians, nurses, and other hospital personnel who treat the mother as a healthy person who is going through a normal process rather than as a sick person who is in danger may facilitate her feelings of competence to care for the child. Further, mothers who are supported psychologically by the caring presence of some person (her mate or some other delivery partner) throughout labor and delivery frequently have less complicated deliveries than mothers who do not experience such support (Klaus & Kennell, 1983).

Perhaps Klaus and Kennell's best known work regarding early influences on bonding is their idea about early parent-child contact and separation. These physician/researchers hypothesize that there is a "maternal sensitive period" during the first minutes and hours after birth when, if parent and child are in contact, interactions can be especially beneficial to the bonding process. Although the existence of such a period is difficult to prove, they believe that early contact increases the parent's confidence, competence, and sensitivity to the infant's crying. "Keeping the mother and baby together soon after birth is likely to initiate and enhance the operation of known sensory, hormonal, physiological, immunological, and behavioral mechanisms that probably attach the parent to the infant" (Klaus & Kennell, 1983, p. 59).

Winnicott (1958) agrees that early contact can be helpful to the development of the parent-child relationship. He believes that early contact helps to relieve the parents' fears that the child may not be healthy or otherwise okay. Klaus and Kennell (1983) also point out that this contact helps the parents to change their mental image of the baby—to replace their fantasy child with the real thing.

While some studies (e.g., Ringler, Kennell, Jarvella, Navojosky, & Klaus, 1975; Ringler, Trause, & Klaus, 1976) have found that early contact is beneficial to the later development of the child, others (e.g., Siegel, 1982) have shown that other factors are even more important. No studies have found early contact to be detrimental to later outcome (Klaus & Kennell, 1983). Early contact can probably be considered helpful, but is neither necessary for, nor sufficient to, the establishment of a bond. In Brazelton's words, ". . . it has become apparent to all of us in the work of supporting parents that bonding initially is not enough [but] . . . the thrill of starting off successfully certainly can enhance one's expectation about being a parent. But it is only one source of energy for attachment" (Klaus & Kennell, 1983, p. ix).

Whatever the factors may be that influence the parents' bond to the child, positive feelings and desire to spend time with the infant characterize this bond. These feelings of love apparently enhance parent-child interaction and have a positive influence on the child's experience of the family context.

Separation/Individuation

The second idea, often called separation/individuation, relates to the child's development of a sense of self as a unique being, separate from, but related to, other people. This process runs parallel to that of attachment and often seems to be a slightly different view of the same events and interactions. Both ideas have been developed with emphasis on the child's relationship to the mother, but may also be used to understand the child's interactions with other caregivers.

In the words of Deutsch (1945), "Woman's two greatest tasks as a mother are to shape her unity with the child in a harmonious manner and later to dissolve it harmoniously" (p. 294). The parallel tasks of the child are to maintain a physically and psychologically necessary unity with the mother and then as the child becomes able to function independently, to differentiate from his or her mother and to become a separate and autonomous individual.

The process through which the mother and child strive to attain these goals early in their relationship have been considered by many authors. Erikson (1963) speaks of the child's development of a sense of confidence that the mother will be there for him or her as "basic trust." He states, "The infant's first social achievement, then, is his willingness to let the mother out of sight without undue anxiety or rage, because she has become an inner certainty as well as an outer predictability" (p. 247). This trust, according to Erikson, depends not on quantities of food given, or on other tangible things, but ". . . rather on the quality of the maternal relationship" (p. 249).

The theory of separation/individuation views the tie between parents and child from a different vantage point than that of attachment theory; it focuses on the child's developing sense of separateness rather than on the bond. Mahler, who developed this theory during years of observation of parents (particularly mothers) and children, refers to this process of developing awareness as the "psychological birth of the individual" (Mahler, Pine, & Bergman, 1975, p. 3). She interprets separation and individuation as ". . . two complementary developments: separation consists of the child's emergence from a symbiotic fusion with the mother . . . and individuation consists of those achievements marking the child's assumption of his own individual characteristics" (Mahler et al., 1975, p. 4). While these processes are never really finished, the most intensive work on them is completed during the period between approximately the 5th and 36th months of life (Mahler et al., 1975).

In contrast to Bowlby's view that the child very slowly becomes tied or attached to the mother at some time after the age of six months, Mahler considers the child and mother to exist, at least in the child's perception, as a "dual unity" much earlier than that, between the second and sixth months. At about five months the child begins to "hatch" from that unity, and to move progressively away from the mother in the process of realizing his or her separateness and developing a sense of self (Mahler, 1968).

The Developmental Process of Early Relationships

Brazelton and Cramer (1990) organize the progression of early interaction into four stages: (1) homeostatic control, (2) prolonging of attention, (3) testing limits, and (4) emergence of autonomy. Their somewhat eclectic view of development includes information from many researchers and from different schools of thought. In this section, early interaction will be discussed using Brazelton and Cramer's stages as well as information on attachment/bonding and separation/individuation. In all of these stages, the baby and his or her caregivers are considered to be participating in bidirectional, transactional interactions; both of their contributions to the development of interaction are considered.

Stage I: *Homeostatic Control (The First Week to Ten Days of Life)*

During this first stage of adaptation, babies have to be able to achieve control over "their input and output systems" in order to pay attention to their caregivers

(Brazelton & Cramer, 1990, p. 113). To do this, they must be able to screen out or receive incoming stimuli while maintaining control over their physiological system and state of consciousness (see Chapter 7 for more information on infant states of consciousness). This is a difficult task and babies need the help of caregivers to accomplish it.

The caregiver's role in helping the infant to gain homeostatis is to allow the baby to gain control and be comfortable in attending by adjusting the amount of input to a level that does not under- or overstimulate the baby. This requires a great deal of empathy and sensitivity on the part of the parent (Brazelton & Cramer, 1990).

Brazelton and Cramer (1990) report that in the normal infant this level of control can be achieved in the first week to ten days of life. For infants with impairments and their caregivers it may be a more difficult, time-consuming task.

Stage II: *Prolonging of Attention (One to Eight Weeks)*

During the second stage, infants "begin to attend to and use social cues to prolong their states of attention" (Brazelton & Cramer, 1990, p. 114). The social cues which become especially important during this time are smiles, vocalizations, facial expressions, and movements—early communication behaviors. Babies use these behaviors to signal their receptiveness to interaction and to elicit responses from the adult (Brazelton & Cramer, 1990).

The caregivers facilitate this process by becoming aware of the baby's rhythms and learning to synchronize their behavior to the baby's. They let the baby take a break when he or she looks away, for example, and they learn to increase stimulation at times (e.g., increasing pitch variations, or adding a new sound to vocalizations) to engage the baby for a longer period of time. They also imitate the baby's behaviors, providing the first step in teaching the baby to imitate (Brazelton & Cramer, 1990).

In this way primary caregivers, usually mothers, develop a close relationship with their babies. This is the beginning of what Mahler (1968) calls "normal symbiosis." This stage begins between the fourth and sixth week of life and Mahler believes that the infant has no awareness of the mother's separateness from him or herself or of her ability to leave. In this symbiotic phase the infant begins to learn through experience. Memory traces are established and pleasure and need gratification become linked with the mother. Soon a "specific smiling response" for mother, the symbiotic partner, appears and symbiosis is thought to be at its height. By the end of this symbiotic period the infant has acquired two things: "a relatedness which binds him to the commonplace details of life *and* a capacity to re-create the illusion of perfect harmony and bliss" (Kaplan, 1978, p. 90).

During the phase of normal symbiosis, baby and caregiver develop increasing skill in communicating with one another. They educate each other with "mutual cuing." The mother develops skills in holding and regulating the infant who, in turn, develops nonverbal routines that involve, among other things, body molding (adjusting to the contours of the partner's body) and stiffening (Kaplan, 1978).

According to Bowlby (1969), babies are in the first stage of developing attachment from birth to roughly 8 or 12 weeks. During this time babies orient toward any person in their vicinity. This orienting behavior includes ". . . tracking movements of the eyes, grasping and reaching, smiling and babbling" (p. 266). Sometimes babies react to the sight of a face or sound of a voice by ceasing to cry. These behaviors are likely to increase the amount of time that they remain in contact with a given companion. During this phase babies display orienting behavior without discriminating who the figure is; mother is at first no more important than anyone else.

Taking these theories together we get a picture of a baby who is learning to attend to cues and to signal his or her willingness to interact. He or she may attempt to use the behaviors that are developing with any available person, but usually has more success with the primary caregiver who is strongly motivated and sensitive to the infant's capacities for interaction. This sensitivity aids in the development of a special relationship between the infant and the primary caregiver.

Stage III: *Testing Limits (Three and Four Months)*

During this stage, both the caregiver and the infant test and try to extend the infant's abilities to "take in and respond to information" and to "withdraw and recover in a homeostatic system" (Brazelton & Cramer, 1990, p. 116). Baby and caregiver develop playful routines or games in which they learn to mirror each other's style of playing (Stern, 1985). These games are in the form of mutually imitated series of behaviors such as smiling, vocalizing, and moving. As their skill at playing with each other for longer and longer periods of time increases, caregiver and baby should experience a sense of mastery and joy related to the interaction. This sense of joy signals the "goodness of fit" between a baby and partner. If it is absent it may be a sign of problems with the developing relationship (Brazelton & Cramer, 1990).

Research also shows that infants express emotion and respond to emotion expressed by their caregivers. Tronick (1989) characterizes the infant's emotional or "affective" communication behaviors as being "other-directed regulatory behaviors" and "self-directed regulatory behaviors" (p. 113). Other-directed regulatory behaviors, such as crying, reaching, or looking toward a desired object, function to regulate the behavior of someone other than the infant. These behaviors are first seen in the early months of life and are not necessarily intentional. Self-directed regulatory behaviors, such as looking away or thumb sucking, function to control and change the infant's own state.

These expressions allow the infant and caregiver to mutually respond and regulate their interactions as in the dialogue discussed earlier. Tronick (1989) suggests that children develop in a healthy or positive way when their experiences with these emotional interchanges are characterized by coordinated, mutually adapted interactions with the caregiver. Development may be emotionally less healthy when interactions are frequently frustrating, poorly coordinated, or when negative affect predominates.

The optimal result of the mutual attunement that is gained during this period is a rich, mutually satisfying pattern of interaction in which the needs of both participants are met. According to Mahler et al. (1975), the infant who is still in the stage of "normal symbiosis" is very much at one with the caregiver during this time, but their unity is not an aware attachment. It is an attachment based on goodness-of-fit of interaction behaviors and the infant's lack of awareness that the caregiver is a separate being. If nothing happens to upset this unity, the infant will never become a person in his own right. The infant must "hatch" from the comfortable egg of this symbiotic relationship to become a psychological entity, separate from the caregiver.

Bowlby (1969) has found that at about 12 weeks of age the intensity of the infant's friendly responses increases and phase two of attachment begins. During the second phase, which lasts from approximately 12 weeks to six months, the baby continues his friendly behavior toward people. The major difference lies in the child's reaction to his mother. Mother (or any other primary caregiver) is singled out for special displays of smiling, grasping, etc. She is clearly distinguished from others in the environment.

For all of these theorists, the period of time when the infant is three to four months of age is a special time of unity and happiness between the baby and the primary caregiver. They have developed their dialogue skills and have forged a strong foundation for building communication abilities.

Stage IV: *Emergence of Autonomy (Four to Five Months)*

In the next month, a change takes place in the interaction between infant and caregiver. The infant becomes a more independent participant in the interaction. When the parents or other primary caregivers can allow or encourage the baby to initiate or lead the interaction and to explore objects on his or her own, a new dimension is added to the interaction. During this time the baby's cognitive awareness increases as object permanence (the idea that objects continue to exist even when they are not in view) begins. The baby becomes aware of the parents' presence and absence and begins to cry for attention.

When the baby engages in game sequences with the parents, he or she may tune them in and out and thereby control the interaction (Brazelton & Cramer, 1990). Brazelton and Cramer cite the following example of interaction during this time:

> A mother and baby boy sit facing each other: the baby gives a smile or a facial response to her gently initiated overtures. She smiles back appreciatively. They lock onto each other in a brief (10-15 seconds) set of responses. There is a recognition of each other's rhythms of movement, of attentional involvement. This is then *broken* by the baby. He looks away, as if by chance. Often, he will look at one shoe. The parent tries to capture his gaze by increasing her cues. The baby looks past her at the other shoe. She tries to get into his line of vision. He adroitly shifts past her to look back at the first shoe. In a sequence as long as three minutes, he is in control for the major part of it, leading her back and forth while he examines each shoe. When she gives up to look away, he will snap back to focus on her face and recapture her. Within the safety of their interaction, he has practiced his developing but still fragile autonomy. (p. 118)

Brazelton and Cramer point out that some parents may find this stage very difficult because they cannot readily control the baby's behavior. This lack of control may challenge the parents' feelings of competence.

This is the period that Mahler (1968) has labeled as "hatching," the first step in the actual process of separation/individuation. The beginning of the hatching process, which is called the subphase of differentiation, extends from about 5 months to 10 or 11 months of age. During this first subphase the infant emerges from the "symbiotic membrane." This development is brought about by the child's investigations of the environment including the caregivers. As the child explores self, others, and objects and remembers and compares, he or she apparently becomes aware of differences in feelings and sights. These perceptions lead to a dawning awareness of separateness.

In the last stage of Brazelton and Cramer's system, the parent-child relationship has gone beyond the first signs of love and attunement and into the arena of first differences. The interactional basis for communication is presented with its first challenges to the harmony of purpose experienced by most infants and parents up to this point. It is probably from these and later challenges that the need to communicate grows most strongly. If parents and children always agreed and were closely tuned-in to each other there would be no need to go beyond the games of the first few months. As they develop a different focus of attention, different purposes, and desires and lose their physical closeness (due to the baby's motor development) and symbiotic attunement, communication about these differences becomes important to their continued satisfaction with each other.

Later Development (Six Months to Three Years)

Because of the importance of later developments to communication growth, further information will be presented here on the continuing progression of the parent-child interaction as perceived by Mahler and Bowlby. A few months after Brazelton and Cramer's Stage IV, at around seven or eight months, the baby's outward-directed attention leads him or her to perceptually investigate outside objects and people and to "check-back" with the mother as a point of orientation. The baby examines the nonmother people and compares them with the mother. It is at this time that what Spitz (1965) refers to as "eight-month anxiety" or "stranger anxiety" appears. The investigating child realizes that he or she is viewing people who are "not mother" and becomes anxious because mother is "gone."

In the next period of development, which Mahler calls the practicing period, children become intoxicated with their attempts at mastery of locomotor skills. They seem driven to learn to walk and to investigate their environment. This "love affair with the world" (Greenacre, 1971) leads them away from the mother to explore by themselves. They check back with her occasionally, but appear to be assured that she would not leave them.

Soon the toddler's blissful sojourns are disrupted by the dawning realization that mother is very much a separate being who can come and go at will. In conjunction with this realization of her separateness, children renew their interest in mother. Toddlers seek more contact with mother and are sometimes reluctant to be without her. During this period of "rapprochement" children can no longer totally believe in their own omnipotence, and they enter a period of increased awareness of their vulnerability. Their attempts to recontact the mother take on a new form. They approach her with toys, gestures, and words, making contact on a higher, sharing level.

Given a normal progression through the preceding subphases children eventually enter the period of object constancy. In this period, which extends from around three years on, children attain a mental representation of their mother which they can call up from memory even when they are separated from her. This allows them to function autonomously as long as there is no undue stress.

Bowlby also observes that at some time between 6 and 12 months the child becomes increasingly discriminating in his or her choices of people to respond to in a friendly manner. When the mother leaves, the baby attempts to follow her and/or cries in an attempt to remain with her. When she returns, he or she greets her and uses her as a base from which to explore the world. During this period, which Bowlby has labeled phase three of attachment, the child is said to be truly attached and his or her behavior toward the mother becomes organized on a "goal-corrected basis," the goal apparently being to maintain proximity to the mother. Phase three continues through the second year and probably into the third year of life.

In phase four the child begins to acquire ". . . insight into his mother's feelings and motives" (Bowlby, 1969, p. 268). "By observing her behavior and what influences it, a child comes to infer something of his mother's set goals and something of the plans she is adopting to achieve them" (p. 267). At this time the mother and child have formed a "goal-corrected partnership." Bowlby states that he can only ". . . guess at what age [this partnership] begins. It is difficult to believe it does so commonly before a child's second birthday, and for many children it seems likely to be much nearer or after their third" (p. 268).

Bowlby concludes that the "pattern of attachment" differs for each mother and child. "By the time the first birthday is reached both mother and infant have commonly made so many adjustments in response to one another that the resulting pattern of interaction has already become highly characteristic" (p. 347). This pattern becomes stable and both partners exert pressure to maintain it. When the pattern is a favorable one, its stability ". . . is its strength" (p. 349); when it is unfavorable for one or both partners this stability can create problems.

Other researchers and theorists have embellished Bowlby's ideas. Ainsworth, for example, contributed significantly to the theory by further delineating attachment behaviors (Ainsworth, 1967) and by developing a technique called "the strange situation," which can be used to measure or classify the child's level of attachment to the caregiver (Ainsworth and Wittig, 1969).

The primary difference between Bowlby's and Mahler's conceptualizations lies in the importance ascribed to the proximity-maintaining behavior of the child. For Bowlby, this is the all-important evidence of the child's attachment to the mother. Mahler, however, sees this behavior as one manifestation of the child's realization of his or her separateness from the mother. The child uses these behaviors until he or she develops a mental representation of the mother that can be called to mind for comfort.

As with attachment/bonding, the parents' experience of the separation/individuation process can color the way the family functions as a communication growth medium. If child and mother have been "out of sync" in their readiness for some phase of this process, problems can arise. For example, a mother who is very comfortable with the close, cuddly, and special relationship she has with her symbiotic infant may experience some reluctance to move on to the differentiation and practicing subphases of separation/individuation. This reluctance may be expressed in subtle changes in her verbal and/or nonverbal interaction with the infant, making the interchange less mutually satisfying.

The next family-related factor that deserves extra attention is the issue of parent-child interaction and its role in language learning.

THE ROLE OF ADULT INPUT IN LANGUAGE ACQUISITION

Early Interaction and Communication

Language acquisition appears to be largely dependent upon the child's social experience. Recent research into fetal abilities and development (Begly, 1991) supports Verny and Kelly's (1981) argument that communicative interaction begins *in utero*. Additionally, the recognition of the importance of nonverbal communication has allowed researchers and theorists to view the young infant as an active participant in the communication process.

Condon and Sander (1974) found that neonates as young as three days old moved in synchrony with adult speech. They interpreted their findings to mean that infants participate nonverbally in language from virtually the day they are born.

However early it may begin, nonverbal communication seems to "set the stage" for verbal communication. In what has been called a "dialogue of action 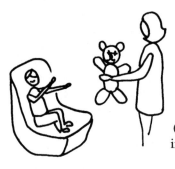 and reaction" (Spitz, 1965), which was discussed earlier in this chapter, infants and caregivers learn to adapt to each other's preferences, to signal for and to maintain attention. Thus, the earliest communication is affective (emotion based) (Thoman, 1981) and leads to a mutually adapted style of interaction unique to each infant-caregiver dyad. Bruner (1977) has emphasized the importance of the infant's and caregiver's joint attention and joint action to the language acquisition process. As the communicative partners learn to read each other's nonverbal indications of attention, a word can readily be associated with the object or action to which it refers.

Early Mother-Child Interaction and Later Cognitive and Language Development

A number of researchers have studied early mother-child interaction as it relates to later child performance. A study of low socioeconomic status infants by Clark-Stewart (1973) found that the mother's verbal stimulation of the child was the single variable most highly related to the child's language competence. Hardy-Brown, Plomin, and DeFries (1981) studied the communicative performance of 50 one-year-old adopted infants and behavioral measures of the birth mother and of the adoptive parents. They found a stronger relationship between infant communication and cognitive ability of the birth mother than the cognitive abilities of the adoptive parents. There were, however, two behaviors of the adoptive mothers which were significantly related to the infant's communicative performance. These were the mother's vocal imitation of the infant and her vocal responsivity to the infant's vocalizations. Olson, Bates, and Bayles (1984) studied mother-infant interaction in 168 dyads. While finding no substantial concurrent relationships between interaction and infant cognitive performance, they did find that maternal verbal stimulation and nurturant physical contact at 6 months of age predicted cognitive competence and language performance at 24 months of age. These studies show that early verbal stimulation and responsiveness to the child appear to be important to both cognitive development and language acquisition.

Language Input to the Language-Learning Child

The characteristics of motherese or child-directed speech have been discussed earlier in this chapter. Once researchers identified the differences between motherese and typical adult-directed speech patterns, speculation began on the actual function of these adaptations for the child. Studies were done which looked at the child's language output and development in response to various forms of adjusted input and other variables of parent-child interaction. An early study by Nelson (1973) showed that language learning was slower when mother and child were not cognitively "matched" and when the mother rejected and/or tried to control the child's verbal output. Other studies found that giving commands and asking too many questions hampered language use, while commenting, reflecting, and expanding the child's utterances facilitated language use (Hetenyi, 1974; Hubbell, 1977; Whitehurst, Novak, & Zorn, 1972). Cross (1978) found that linguistic acquisition was accelerated when: (1) mother's input matched the child's communicative intent; (2) mother used partial repetitions of the child's utterances with expansions and extensions; (3) mother used few utterances new to the discourse; (4) mother's speech was fluent and intelligible; (5) mother used a low level of preverb complexity; and (6) mother used fewer utterances per conversation turn.

Cross (1984) has summarized the literature on this topic, citing research on three general areas of parent input to the child: discourse contingencies; sentence types and associated functions; and input parameters.

Discourse Contingencies

The following parent language behaviors frequently have been found to be positively related to language acquisition: (1) semantic contingency, when the parent's utterance takes the topic of the child's preceding utterance or nonverbal communication; and (2) acknowledgment, when the parent gives a positive/accepting response to the child's utterance.

One parental discourse behavior was found to be negatively related to language growth. This behavior, parental self-repetition, occurs when the parent repeats his or her own utterances.

Sentence Types and Associated Function

Both of the following parent behaviors were negatively related to language growth in studies cited by Cross: (1) imperatives, when the parent uses commands; and (2) questions, when parents used fewer yes/no questions and more wh-questions.

One sentence type, declaratives, was found to be positively related to language growth.

Input Parameters

The amount of speech directed to the child and increased intelligibility and fluency were found to be positively related to language growth. Increased rate of speech to the child was found in four studies to be negatively related to language growth.

Dunst, Lowe, and Bartholomew (1990) argue that contingent social responsiveness (e.g., semantic contingency) of the family to the infant is of such importance to the development of communicative competence that treatment programs should focus on promoting and facilitating this aspect of interaction.

CONCLUSION

This chapter considered the role of the family environment in child language acquisition. It discussed several theoretical views of the importance of that environment, the way the family works as a medium for communication growth, and some of the family-related factors that may influence development. Chapter 3 will look at the family in relationship to communication disorders, the factors that put a child at risk for disorders, and the impact of problems on the family system.

3

The Family and Communication Disorders

Even as families provide a nurturing context for the development of communication, they also are the setting for factors that create risks for communication disorders. Organic and environmental/behavioral conditions that may be present in, or influenced by, the environment may play a role in the development of communication disorders.

WHAT PUTS A CHILD AT RISK FOR COMMUNICATION DISORDERS?

There are many conditions and factors that place a young child at risk for the development of a communication disorder. The term *at risk* indicates that a person has "the potential to develop a disorder based on specific biological, environmental, or behavioral factors" (American Speech-Language-Hearing Association, 1988, p. 90). The conditions or factors that create risk for communication disorders are the same conditions that create risk for many other developmental disorders. Communication disorders are frequently seen in combination with, or as a result of, more general or pervasive developmental problems. Rossetti (1986) has captured the ubiquitous nature of risk factors with the following quote, ". . . anything that interferes with an infant's ability to interact normally with its environment is a potential source of developmental delay" (p. 2).

Estimates of the prevalence of disabling conditions in children in the United States vary depending upon the criteria used. Of the 3.5 million children born in the United States every year, approximately 2 percent, or 70,000 children, have some kind of disabling condition (Healy, 1983). Dinno (1977) reports that 6 percent of all persons in the United States have developmental disorders that are present at birth or in early life. The U.S. Centers for Disease Control (Thacker, 1988) estimate that four million people suffer from some kind of developmental disability at a cost of $16.5 billion per year to federal, state, and private sources.

These numbers, although almost too large to be readily comprehensible, illustrate the importance of early preventive intervention. The monetary cost of disabilities is staggering. Perhaps even more important, but less easily illustrated, is the cost of these conditions in terms of human potential. Disabilities can result in decreased happiness and productivity, and reductions in other contributions to society.

Perinatal Biological Risk Factors and Later Outcome

A great deal of attention has been paid to perinatal biological risk factors such as premature birth and their role in predicting the developmental outcome for high-risk children. It seems only logical that children with significant physical problems at birth (e.g., preterm delivery, respiratory distress syndrome, intracranial hemorrhage) have a greater chance of developmental deviancy than children who have no such problems. However, Sameroff (1982), whose transactional model of development was discussed in Chapter 2, reports that significant relationships have not been found between perinatal risk factors and later outcome except where there is also an environmental risk such as poverty. He identifies the "caretaking environment" as the deciding factor in such cases. A "sufficiently supportive and adaptive" environment can compensate for almost any biological condition. He states:

> It has become increasingly clear that what we have previously thought to be characteristics of the child that are independent of child rearing context are inextricably tied to the experiential environment. Only the most extreme cases of brain damage still present us with immutable children. . . . Variations in experience produce variation in outcome . . . individual plasticity is a consequence of contextual plasticity. (p. 151)

It seems that whatever the biological condition of the child, the transactional process that occurs in the environment plays an important role in determining developmental outcome. The quality of caregiving in that environment is apparently of paramount importance. There seem to be specific characteristics of the caregiving environment that determine whether it will be able to compensate for biological insult. Moreover, there may be some environments that fail to compensate for even the most minor risk, or that actually create risk.

After studying the effects of developmental risk factors, Sameroff (1982) concluded:

> At one end of the continuum the caretaking environment was sufficiently supportive and adaptive to compensate for almost any biologi-

cal risk factor so that it was not transformed into later intellectual or emotional problems. At the other end of the continuum the caretaking environment had neither the educational, emotional, nor economic resources to deal with even minor perinatal problems. Thus, the child, if allowed to survive, would maintain deficits into later stages of intellectual and emotional growth. (p. 142)

Sameroff (1975, 1982) has used his transactional model to explain the relationship between early risk factors and later developmental outcome of the child. Using this model as a structure, we can gain some insight into the different experiences of children and parents from different families. For example, Jeremy, a newborn with a cleft lip and palate, was taken home to a modest but comfortable suburban home by his parents, Marie and John Taylor. The Taylors have two older children, five and nine years of age, who are developing normally. Although the Taylors were initially shocked by Jeremy's appearance, sensitive professionals helped them to understand the operations and procedures that would be done to correct the facial and palatal defects. They also helped Marie to learn to feed Jeremy with a special nipple. Using a transactional point of view, we can trace one of the early interactions for this family:

Child Transaction

1. Jeremy (J) cries and roots, indicating that he is hungry.

2. J takes the nipple and begins to feed. Some liquid is regurgitated through his nose.

3. J feeds well for several minutes. He meets his mother's gaze for several seconds at a time. He falls asleep after being burped.

Parent Transaction

1. Marie (M) prepares a bottle confidently as she would have for her other children, but uses the adapted nipple that works best for J. She picks J up and holds him comfortably, feeling his responses to different postures.

2. M removes the nipple, says, "Oh my, that was hard for you. Let's try holding your head up a little higher and see if that helps." She adjusts J's position and begins to feed him again, smiling and gaining eye contact with her baby.

3. M holds her sleeping baby, reflecting on his differences from her older children and on the challenges he presents to her mothering abilities. She places him in his cradle and goes about her next task of feeding the older children.

Another child, Harold, was also born with a cleft lip and palate. His mother, Sharon, is a single, 17-year-old high school senior who lives with her parents in a two-bedroom trailer in a rural area. When Harold was born, the medical personnel quickly cleaned him up and took him to the nursery without showing him to Sharon. They told her simply, "Your baby has a problem." Sharon and her parents were very upset when they finally saw Harold. The nursing staff explained what could be done to correct Harold's defects and showed Sharon and her mother how to feed him. Sharon heard little of what they said. We can trace Sharon's interactions with Harold:

Child Transactions	*Parent Transactions*
1. Harold (H) cries and roots, indicating that he is hungry.	1. Sharon (S) picks H up gingerly, letting his head fall back.
2. H's cries intensify.	2. S sits down and puts H on her lap, facing her. She gazes at him, wondering why she has had such an ugly baby. She jiggles her knees a bit and says, "Hush now. Crying ain't gonna make you look any better."
3. H cries louder.	3. S calls to her mother, "Ma, I don't know what's wrong with this baby. He just keeps crying." S puts H back in his crib and turns the radio up louder.

The differences between the experiences of these two infants and parents are clear. One can guess at the different developmental processes that they will follow, and at the dissimilarity in their developmental outcome.

Research by Escalona (1982) supports the idea of the environment's influence on development. Her findings indicate that a stressful or deficient environment is especially detrimental for preterm infants.

To further investigate these issues, Menyuk, Liebergott, Schultz, Chesnick, and Ferrier (1991) followed a group of preterm infants and a group of full-term infants for three years. They found that the preterm infants' lexical and cognitive development was not markedly different from that of the group of full-term infants. Only a subgroup of very low birth weight (VLBW) infants (less than 1500 grams in weight) differed significantly from the full-term infants on two measures. Even given the differences, the scores of these VLBW infants were within normal limits. Menyuk et al. speculate that the lack of differences may be attributed to the fact that none of their subjects was chronically ill or came from impoverished families. In addition, the experimental procedure itself, which called for the mothers to keep diaries of their children's language use and for monthly visits by professionals to collect data, may have enhanced language development of all of the children. Findings of this study appear to support Sameroff's contention that favorable environmental conditions may mitigate early biological risks.

Among the many factors that influence the transactions between the child and the environment are the child's own "self-righting tendencies." As long as the environment provides the opportunity for interaction, the child tends to compensate for deficits and to develop necessary skills. Sameroff (1982) cites the example of the thalidomide babies who, despite lack of limbs, achieved the aspects of normal cognitive development that most infants achieve by eye-hand coordination, for example, by coordinating whatever they had (that is, if functional hands were not available, they coordinated their feet or some other body part).

The transactional model is similar to the "interactionist model" of development proposed by Ramey and Baker-Ward (1982). These authors point out that heredity and environment operate to create a phenotype, the resulting expression of genetic programming. They argue that while the early experiences of children are important to development, later experiences also have important effects. These effects may be positive or negative. "If the quality of the fostering environment improves during the life span, the debilitating effects of early adversity can be mitigated. Similarly, if the environment becomes less supportive, early developmental gains can be lost" (p. 284).

EXERCISE #1

Think about the "fostering environment" of children or adults you know who were born prematurely or with some other perinatal biological risk factor (check the list in the following section for other risk factors). Can you think of any whose experiences seem to have helped them develop in an especially positive way? What factors do you think were particularly important to their development? How do you think they may have contributed to the interactions with their caregivers?

Risk Factors

Despite the influence of the environment and later experience on the ultimate outcome for high-risk infants, it is important to recognize the factors or conditions that place a child at risk for the development of communication disorders. It is especially important that we recognize these risk factors because infants and toddlers who are at risk are eligible for services under P.L. 99-457 (see Chapter 1) if states choose to include them in the system. The risk factors can be divided into two broad categories, organic factors and environmental/behavioral factors.

These categories are not necessarily mutually exclusive; some factors belong under both headings. The risk factors are listed below, followed by examples and other criteria for inclusion in a high-risk registry or tracking system. Some of the criteria are drawn from Blackman (1986). The presence of any of these risk factors, especially two or more factors in combination, in an infant or toddler's history should serve as a red flag that alerts us to monitor the development of communication abilities.

Organic Factors (Intrinsic to the Child)

1. *Genetic disorders* that lead to abnormal growth and development or specific communication problems. For example:

- chromosomal disorders such as Down syndrome or Fragile X syndrome
- hearing loss due to genetic disorders
- cleft lip and/or palate
- single gene disorders such as tuberous sclerosis or Williams syndrome

2. *Congenital disorders and other conditions related to prenatal development* that may lead to structural, developmental, and/or functional deficits include

- lack of prenatal care
- maternal phenylketonuria
- maternal use of therapeutic drugs such as anticonvulsants
- parental substance abuse
- microcephaly, macrocephaly, or other central nervous system abnormality
- hyperbilirubinemia
- maternal diabetes
- cleft lip and/or palate

3. *Low birth weight* (less than 2000 grams), especially very low birth weight (less than 1500 grams), which leads to general vulnerability. Low birth weight can occur due to

- prematurity
- intrauterine growth retardation

4. *Perinatal problems* related to damage of the neonate and development of conditions such as cerebral palsy include

- respiratory distress
- asphyxia
- intracranial hemorrhage
- neonatal seizures

5. *Illness, accidents, or abuse* that lead to structural or functional deficits. For example

- maternal AIDS
- anemia
- central nervous system (CNS) insult due to conditions such as
  —infection (e.g., STORCH [the acronym for syphilis, toxoplasmosis, other infections, rubella, cytomegalic inclusion disease, and herpes], meningitis)
  —trauma
  —toxin (e.g., lead)
  —metabolic disorder
  —asphyxia
  —CNS malignancy
- severe chronic illness such as
  —respiratory problems
  —renal disease
  —chronic otitis media
  —seizure disorder

6. *Iatrogenic disorders* (i.e., disorders caused by treatment) such as

- vocal fold damage due to intubation
- hearing loss due to ototoxic drugs

Environmental/Behavioral Factors

1. *Poverty and inadequate living conditions* may include

- unsanitary/unsafe environment (hazards, pollution, toxins)
- lack of permanent housing
- excessively noisy environment

2. *Psychosocial factors* such as

- deficient parent-child attachment
- lack of support systems (social, financial, emotional)
- inappropriate caregiver expectations
- insensitivity to child needs and capacities

3. *Deficient caregiver competence* (physical, intellectual, educational, emotional) due to conditions such as

- maternal age of less than 18 years
- parental sensory impairment
- parental mental retardation
- parental mental illness

4. *Caregiver behaviors* that fail to provide adequate conditions for communication development may include

- disordered parenting (abuse or neglect of the child)
- over- or understimulation
- high percentage of negative/rejecting/directive responses to child behaviors (especially communication behaviors)
- inadequate language model (form, content, use, rate)

This list illustrates the broad range of factors that can influence communication development. Sometimes the conditions related to risk factors are obvious and have an immediate impact on the child, and sometimes they are less apparent. When the risk is based on a condition that impairs the child's abilities, the effects of this impairment are often felt on the family as well as the child.

THE IMPACT OF IMPAIRMENT ON THE FAMILY

The World Health Organization has labeled the progressive consequences of diseases and disorders as *impairment, disability,* and *handicap.* An impairment is a "loss or abnormality of psychological, physiological or anatomical structure or function" (Wood, 1980, p. 376). Disability refers to a reduced ability to meet the needs of daily living, and handicap denotes the societal disadvantage, due to an impairment and resulting disability, that an individual experiences.

The degree of handicap depends on the attitudes and biases of those who are in contact with the disabled individual (Beukelman, 1986). For the purposes of this book we will consider the infant who has a condition that can lead to a handicap to be impaired and at-risk for developing a disability and resulting handicap, rather than *ipso facto* handicapped. These infants are at risk for developing a disability and resulting handicap, but are not necessarily "handicapped infants" or in many cases even "infants with disabilities."

Initial Reaction to an Impairment

Infants who are born with an obvious biological risk factor that is apparent from the time of birth may create a special condition within the family into which they are born. Parents-to-be often dream of an idealized baby who is close to perfect and who fulfills all of their needs and expectations. This is not to say that expectant parents never consider the possibility of having an impaired baby. In fact, Brazelton (1983) reports that parents-to-be often imagine many different things that might go wrong and "rehearse for a damaged infant" (p. viii). This turmoil often seems to serve the purpose of mobilizing the parents' energy to adjust to parenthood and to bond with their baby (Brazelton, 1983, p. viii).

For the parents whose fears are realized by the birth of an impaired child, there are often feelings of shock and disappointment or at very least a violation of their expectations of that perfect, need-fulfilling baby. For example, when a low birth weight child is born, its early arrival, appearance, unusual cry, unnatural feeding procedures and conditions under which interaction can take

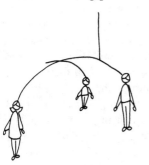

place (with life-saving devices such as the isolette, intravenous tubes, nasogastric tubes, etc.), and slow developmental progress all violate the parents' expectations of what should occur with a baby (Parke & Tinsley, 1982). The parents' unmet expectations may bring about a state of disequilibrium in their relationship or in the whole family (Parke & Tinsley, 1982) at a time which is stressful under the best of circumstances.

A number of factors have been found to affect the parents' reaction to the birth of an impaired child or to the diagnosis of a risk-related condition in a child not previously known to be impaired. One such factor is the manner in which the parents are informed of the condition (Meyer, 1986; Mori, 1983; Price-Bonham & Addison, 1978; Simpson, 1982). This factor is said to affect both the parents' later relationships with professionals (Simpson, 1982) and their "adjustment to and acceptance of the child" (Price-Bonham & Addison, 1978, p. 223). Ehly, Conoley, and Rosenthal (1985) report that there are many potential problems with the manner in which professionals inform parents of their child's impairment. These include

- delay in defining the problem
- false encouragement of parents
- too much advice on matters such as institutionalization
- abruptness
- hurriedness
- lack of interest
- hesitancy to communicate (p. 16)

Other factors that reportedly affect the parents' reactions include the severity of the possible handicap, the social acceptability of the handicap, the socioeconomic status (SES) of the family (with higher and lower SES families being variously reported to react more adversely), and the age at which the child is diagnosed (Mori, 1983). While many factors can exacerbate or mitigate the parents' reaction, there are apparently no factors that insulate parents from the grieving process which is a commonly reported reaction to the loss of the dreamed-of-perfect baby.

One other factor that should probably be noted concerning the parental reaction to a child's impairment is the parents' ability status. For example, some deaf parents are reportedly relieved and pleased to give birth to a deaf child because a deaf child will fit more readily into the deaf culture of which the parents are a part (S. Cooper, personal communication, April 1989).

The emotional adjustment that most parents must make when their child is diagnosed as having a significant problem or impairment has frequently been likened to the stages of grief experienced with death and dying (Mori, 1983; Simpson, 1982). Kubler-Ross's (1969) model in which the dying or people whose loved ones die pass through five stages (denial and isolation; anger; bargaining; depression; and acceptance) is often used to explain the parental response to diagnosis. Another feeling which is common to the parents of these children is guilt. Parents frequently believe, correctly or incorrectly, that something they did caused the child's condition.

Gargiulo (1984) reports that parents pass through three stages as they adjust to the child's condition. In the first phase, parents feel shock and disbelief, denial, grief, and depression. In the second phase, guilt becomes a major factor. At this time parents may also feel ambivalence, and later, anger with questions such as "Why me?" In the third phase parents may bargain, adapt and reorganize, and finally accept the child's status.

Gargiulo points out, however, that these stages should not be seen as rigidly fixed or as proceeding in only one direction. The stages are fluid and parents may move back and forth as they adapt. Gargiulo further notes that not all parents will reach a state of acceptance; many parents will always feel some degree of pain, sorrow, and disappointment. Both Simpson (1982) and Meyer (1986) report that parents often experience "chronic sorrow" throughout the child's life.

Mori (1983) found that parents of impaired children pass through three stages as they react to the child's diagnosis. In Mori's early stage, parents experience "severe psychological disorganization" and they are often "overwhelmed and frantic" (p. 21) with feelings of shock, hopelessness, and self-pity. During the middle stages, parents frequently reject the diagnosis and "shop" for different causes and/or cures. In the final stage, parents gain acceptance based on reality.

In *The Broken Cord,* Dorris (1989) writes of his struggles to understand and deal with the developmental problems of his adopted son, Adam, who was eventually diagnosed as having fetal alcohol syndrome. He expresses many feelings that parents of infants and toddlers with disabilities may have.

> Up until Adam was almost seven, while he was a first and only child, there was no basis for comparison. I strove to accept uncritically his unique developmental schedule as appropriate. He was the product of so many special circumstances, so many adverse factors, that I publicly persisted in my defensive optimism long after a sense of dread had entered my nightly dreams.
>
> As time passed I blamed racism: negative evaluators underrated Adam because of unconscious, unexpressed negative feelings about minorities. I discounted as "culture biased" the IQ tests that consistently scored my son in the upper sixties or low seventies. I periodically concluded that Adam's teachers must be incompetent, badly trained, or lazy when they failed to stimulate his performance in the classroom. I protested haughtily to principals, counselors, even, on one occasion, to the federal government. (p. 75)

Luterman (1991) presents a slightly different point of view of this process which he called the coping process. In his view there are four fluid stages—denial, resistance, affirmation, and integration—which lead to the ability to cope in one way or another. Denial or failure to recognize and deal directly with a problem or the objective signs of a problem is seen as a normal reaction to feelings of inadequacy. If parents have no other way of dealing with a problem, they may continue to deny its existence.

In the resistance stage, parents recognize the existence of a problem but appear to believe that they can defeat it. They often refuse to join support groups, stubbornly insisting that they can overcome the problem on their own. Luterman reports that parents often have to "hit an emotional bottom" before they can move beyond this stage.

When parents reach the affirmation stage they acknowledge their loss to themselves and to the rest of the world. They often become active in various organizations related to the problem and take on a new identity which includes the problem (Luterman, 1991).

In the integration stage, parents learn to live with the problem and to get on with other things as well. They may develop a lifestyle that allows them to enjoy life fully while coping with the effects of the problem (Luterman, 1991).

There are several means of coping that an individual may adopt. Luterman (1991) cited four: flight (leaving the situation, as in divorce); modification (modifying the disability, as with a hearing aid); reframing (changing the way the situation is viewed, e.g., "It could be worse . . ."); and stress reduction (finding ways to deal with the stress, as with working out, meditating, etc.).

Impact on the Family System

In the first chapter of this book, the family was discussed as a system in which family members held positions and filled roles relative to one another. In this system, family members were seen as working on developmental tasks as the family progressed through various life cycle stages. It was emphasized that as one family member changed, the family system changed in order to maintain some kind of balance. The addition of a new member to a family system is always a stressful event which demands that family roles change and that new developmental tasks be addressed. When that new family member violates family expectations and/or requires an unexpected amount or kind of caregiving, or when his or her health is in jeopardy, the family system is especially vulnerable to disequilibrium. If the family is viewed as a developing system, then the entire family may be at risk for developmental problems when a member is born with, or is discovered to have, a significant impairment.

In Turnbull and Turnbull's (1986) view, the impairment of a family member affects the family resources, family interaction, and family functions in significant ways (see Chapter 1). For example, the characteristics of the impairment, its type, severity, and time of discovery, all impact on the family resources. Likewise, the impairment can affect family interaction by having an impact on the relationships among subsystems of family members. It may put added stress on the mother-father subsystem, create communication problems for the mother-child or father-child subsystem, or change sibling-sibling interaction if the nonimpaired sibling must provide care for the impaired sibling.

These alterations in family resources and family inter-action may change the family functions that result. The function of meeting economic needs may suffer additional stress due to the added medical expenses often encountered with an impaired child, or recre-ational needs may be more difficult to meet because of special requirements of an im-paired family member.

Long-Term Impact on Family Members

The literature on families of children with impairments contains reports of the impact of the impairment on various family mem-bers. Following the initial shock and grief reactions discussed earlier, parents generally regain some sense of equilibrium (Meyer, 1986). It has been noted, however, that both parents may continue to experience disappointment, anger, guilt (Lamb, 1983), or even chronic sorrow (Meyer, 1986). Many factors appear to influence the parents' ability to cope with the impaired child. Both the child's temperament and the parents' relationship with one another influence reactions to and interactions with the child (Mori, 1983; Park & Tinsley, 1982). Parents' reactions may also be influenced by the support system available, the severity of the impairment, and the child's prognosis (Meyer, 1986). In addition, parents may have unrealistic expectations for development of the impaired child. The stress that these expectations cause may contribute to serious parenting difficulty (Park & Tinsley, 1982).

Moroney (1981) lists a number of difficulties faced by parents of children with impairments

- financial problems
- actual or perceived stigma
- time demands for personal care of child
- difficulty with caregiving (feeding, for example)
- decreased time for sleep
- social isolation
- less time for recreation
- difficulty managing behavior
- difficulty with routine household chores
- pessimism about the future

Studies of mothers of impaired children indicate that they may experience difficulty in bonding with the infant, that caregiving may be more difficult, separations due to hospitalizations may disrupt parent-child interaction, and other people's reactions to the child may influence interaction (Ramey, Beckman-Bell, & Gowan, 1980).

Fathers of impaired children may react differently to the condition than do mothers. Mothers reportedly are most concerned with emotional issues and concerns about child care; fathers may be more concerned with economic issues and long-term problems (Lamb, 1983; Meyer, 1986). Lamb (1983) reports that fathers are especially concerned with the visibility of the child's impairment and the child's behavior outside the home. Fathers are also reported to be more concerned if the impaired child is a boy (Lamb, 1983; Meyer, 1986).

The father's role as a caregiver is somewhat more active when a child is impaired. Fewell (1986) and Park and Tinsley (1982) report that fathers are more involved with child care and housework with handicapped and preterm infants in the home.

Of course, mothers and fathers are not the only family members who may be affected by an impaired family member. Siblings of the child may also feel the impact of his or her special needs and abilities. Although much of the information on the effects on siblings is from anecdotal reports rather than carefully designed studies (Crnic & Leconte, 1986), a number of common issues emerge. Siblings commonly fear that they may have caused the problem, or that they or their future children may also be defective (Crnic & Leconte, 1986; Fewell, 1986; Stewart, 1986). Siblings often report negative influences when they are required to accept a large portion of responsibility for the care of an impaired brother or sister (Simpson, 1982; Crnic & Leconte, 1986; Stewart, 1986). This is frequently true when the nonimpaired sibling is an older female (Crnic & Leconte, 1986; Fewell, 1986). Other effects felt by siblings include competition for parent attention and feelings of neglect; need to compensate for the impaired sibling; and confusion and lack of communication about the handicapping condition (Crnic & Leconte, 1986; Stewart, 1986; Simpson, 1982).

The impact of having an impaired sibling is reportedly mediated by responsibility for caregiving; age and birth order; individual temperament; the family's socioeconomic status; and the parents' attitudes (Crnic & Leconte, 1986). Grossman (1972) reported that the parents' attitudes and reactions to retarded siblings were the strongest influences on the siblings' acceptance of the retarded child. Clearly, not all siblings suffer because of an impaired family member (Simpson, 1982).

Yet another group of family members who may feel the impact of an impaired child is the grandparents. Grandparents are often important components of the family's support system. They may provide such help as financial aid, babysitting, friendship, and conflict mediation (Sonneck, 1986). Sonneck reports that grandparents may be less supportive when there is a handicapped child in the family. Gabel and Kotsch (1981) suggest two reasons why this might be true: (1) the grandparents may have a strong reaction to the birth of an impaired child just as the parents do, and have to deal with their own anger and grief; and (2) grandparents may feel inadequate to meet the special needs of an impaired child. When grandparents or other members of the extended family fail to provide the expected support for the family with an impaired child, that family is at even greater risk of having its own developmental difficulties.

Clearly, the impact of many of the conditions that may put a child at risk for communication disorders is felt by many people other than the child. In addition to this breadth of influence, the impact of some conditions, especially more severe impairments, may be especially strong at certain times during the family life cycle or at the time of certain events. The following events or times in early life have been noted as being especially stressful for family members: (1) when the impairment is diagnosed (Fewell, 1986; Meyer, 1986); (2) during early childhood when delays in development and continued need for unusual care become apparent (Fewell, 1986; Meyer, 1986); and (3) at the time of school entry if the child cannot benefit from a regular classroom situation (Fewell, 1986).

Parke and Tinsley (1982) view the at-risk infant as being embedded within a larger social system with several important components: (1) the mother-child-father family system, (2) the formal and informal support systems, and (3) the cultural system.

EXERCISE #2

If it is possible for you to talk with members of the family of some person you know who has a disability, do so. Ask about their experiences shortly after they learned about the disabling condition, how their feelings may have changed over time, how they coped with various aspects of the problem, etc.

If you are not able to talk with an actual family member, search the literature for articles and books about such families, for example:

Berg, B. (1982, April). When it happens to you. *Savvy,* 44-47. This article tells of the experiences of a professional couple whose child was born with Down syndrome.

Miller, S. (1990). *Family pictures.* New York: Harper Collins. This work of fiction chronicles the life of the family of a child with autism.

Dorris, M. (1989). *The broken cord.* New York: Harper & Row. This is a nonfictional account of the author's experience of life with his adopted child with fetal alcohol syndrome which also gives excellent information on the syndrome.

If you do this as a class project, it may be especially interesting to interview or read about families from different cultures and compare their reactions.

IMPACT ON THE FAMILY AS AN EARLY COMMUNICATION CONTEXT

The impaired child develops communication abilities, or fails to develop them, in a language-learning environment that may differ from that available to the unimpaired child. In Chapter 2, the family was described as a context for communication development. It was seen as providing four important inputs to the child's learning of communication: (1) stimuli for development-promoting interaction; (2) conditions that stimulate need and desire for communication; (3) communication/language models and opportunities; and (4) consequences for attempts to communicate.

While the following section is written with the impaired child in mind, some of the conditions described may be equally true for unimpaired children who are born under less-than-optimal conditions. For example, children born into families who are experiencing high levels of stress, who have recently experienced the loss of a member, or who did not desire a child, may experience some of the same conditions that a child with an impairment does. Of course, all families respond differently to impairments, and different impairments elicit different responses. The following comments are necessarily general in nature.

Impact on Stimuli for Development-Promoting Interaction

Newborn infants are usually brought into a world that is busy with people and events. Relatives and friends visit and bring gifts to express their happiness in welcoming the new family member. The baby is the center of joyful attention.

The picture may be different when an impaired, premature, or unhealthy child is born. Friends and relatives may be reluctant to call or visit because they are unsure of what to say or are fearful of upsetting the parents.

One grandmother told the following story in a "Dear Abby" column (*Baltimore Sun,* Oct. 2, 1989):

Dear Abby: Six months ago, our 22-year-old daughter gave birth to her second son. Within hours of the baby's birth, our lives were changed forever. Our beautiful and apparently healthy grandchild has a condition known as Down syndrome. Our grief was almost indescribable for those first weeks following his birth—and was often compounded by thoughtless but well-intentioned comments from friends and relatives.

We were asked, "Which side of the family is to blame?" And the most ignorant question of all: "Are you going to keep him?"

Abby, this baby is special, but not because he is handicapped. We would have loved him just as much had he been born without Down syndrome. Time has eased our grief and enabled us to let go of the dreams and plans we had for this child. New dreams and different plans have taken their place.

The birth of a handicapped baby is traumatic to the family. Friends and relatives can be a source of comfort and strength. They should acknowledge the baby's birth with appropriate gifts, cards, letters, etc., as they would for any other newborn.

If one is in doubt as to what to say, it is best to remain silent. A gentle squeeze of the hand or a warm hug can speak volumes.

The child's early experience may include more attention from medical personnel than interaction with parents. For example, if the child needs care in the neonatal intensive care unit (NICU), contact with the parents immediately after birth may be impossible or very brief. Continued hospitalization under the special conditions of the NICU (with isolettes, monitors, feeding tubes, etc.) may further interfere with normal parent-child interaction. The infant may be cared for by many different people, and the mother and father may have difficulty developing skills as caregivers. It has been argued that these conditions make it more difficult for parents to bond to their sick or low birth weight infant (Klaus & Kennell, 1983).

When the baby does leave the hospital, there may still be fewer relatives and friends around to support the parents than expected under normal circumstances. As noted earlier, even grandparents may feel inadequate to deal with the special needs of an impaired infant and may be less willing than usual to visit or to babysit.

If the parents are grieving, people may be uncomfortable interacting with them and may withdraw. Interactions with people who do come into the home may be strained and filled with tension. Under these circumstances, the early dialogue or nonverbal interchange with the baby may differ from that seen with most healthy babies. Important nonverbal communication behaviors such as eye contact and holding may be limited or deficient in some respect either due to the baby's or parents' behavior.

Contact with professionals may continue to play a role in the family's routine, especially if a follow-up program is necessary. While this involvement may be

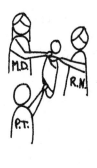

necessary and ultimately helpful, the family may consider it as intruding or interfering with their establishment of a manageable routine.

The physical environment that the infant experiences may be largely restricted to the home, special education center, and medical facility if the child's health is not stable, or if the parents have difficulty with public reactions to the child. In addition, the child's interaction with objects may be limited by a physical or sensory impairment, or by family members who may be "too helpful" to allow the child to learn from frustrating interactions with toys or other objects.

The events that the infant experiences may also be different from those to which most infants are exposed. Daily routines may revolve around visits to various therapists, often to the extent that parents are tired, "hassled," and generally under stress. Special events which normally provide pleasure and relief from routine, such as family parties, visits to the zoo, or vacations, may be restricted due to medical, physical, or social problems.

Clearly, impaired children may be at risk for limited or inadequate interactions with the people and things. Their opportunities for learning about the world and the way it works may be limited, and their perception of their role in that world may differ from that of unimpaired children.

Need and Desire To Communicate

In addition to opportunities to learn about the world, the family provides conditions that produce the motivation or need and desire to communicate. As described in Chapter 2, infants' early use of nonverbal communication typically attracts the caregiver to them and promotes caring interaction. As infants' early attempts at tension reduction through crying, smiling, etc., are interpreted as meaningful communication, they begin to grasp the power of communicative behaviors and to attempt to use them intentionally. The infant-caregiver attachment fuels this process by providing the desire to interact on the part of the caregiver and the infant.

These conditions may be different for the impaired child. The infant's appearance, nonverbal communication, and even his or her cry may differ greatly from what the parents and other family members expected. These differences may make it difficult for caregivers to become attracted to the infant. It may be more difficult to interpret the infant's communication. For example, low birth weight (LBW) infants often engage in behaviors such as startle responses, yawning, or finger splaying when they are overstimulated or otherwise distressed (Als, Lawhorn, Brown, Gibes, Duffy, McAnulty, & Blickman, 1986). Parents who are unaware of the significance of these behaviors may misintrepret or ignore them and consequently increase the stress that the infant experiences.

The feeding situation, which is often prime time for positive interaction and communication, may become an especially difficult time for LBW or impaired infants (Parke & Tinsley, 1982). Hypersensitivity in the oral area or complications in sucking or swallowing may make eating unpleasant for the child, and the parents may become frustrated and experience feelings of inadequacy because of these difficulties.

When such problems occur in very basic interactions, it is easy to see how difficulty with attachment can occur. The process of separation/individuation is also at risk when the child experiences problems with normal development and functioning (Mordock, 1979). If, for example, a motorically impaired child is unable to creep, crawl, or walk, he or she may have difficulty moving beyond the phase of "differentiation" to "practicing." This failure to progress may mean that the child continues to experience the stranger anxiety that is often seen during the earlier phase.

Impact on Communication/Language Models and Opportunities and Consequences of Communication Attempts

The issue of how language input and response may or may not affect language learning in some children is far from a simple one. Conditions related to impairment can interfere with the nonverbal dialogue that develops between caregivers and infants. Because early development of verbal communication is built upon the patterns of interaction laid down in this dialogue, it is reasonable to suspect that the language models provided for some infants may be equally affected. It is important to remember that not only infants with notable impairments may experience these conditions. Many other factors can influence parent-child interaction in similar ways.

Studies comparing the interaction of normal language-learning children and their parents with interaction of parent-child dyads where the child is language disordered have been done. These studies of parent-child interaction are far from uniform in their findings, but there are some recurring themes which run through many of them. Some parent behaviors appear to facilitate child communication, while others appear to constrain it. For example, contingent responding (responses that maintain the child's topic of conversation) by the parents has been shown to be positively related to child communication ability, while negative or nonaccepting responding and directiveness by the parents have been shown to be negatively related to child communication ability

(Bondurant, Romeo, & Kretschmer, 1983; Cross, 1984; Wulbert, Inglis, Kreigsman, & Mills, 1975).

Two treatment-oriented studies of parent interaction with language-disordered children have shown that parents can be helped to develop communication behaviors that are apparently more facilitative of language development (Tiegerman & Siperstien, 1984), and that mothers do appear to change the nature of their verbal interactions with the child as the child's language ability improves (Price, 1983).

Despite the evidence from these studies, the relationship between parent input and child behaviors has become a controversial issue for a number of reasons. There has been a failure to replicate findings from study to study. Studies have frequently assumed that parent behaviors caused child deficits; it is also possible that child deficits lead to parent behavioral change, bringing about the differences that are seen between parents of language-normal children and children with disordered language. In addition, there have been many methodological difficulties with the studies. For example, the number of subjects have generally been few, the definitions of "language impaired" have lacked uniformity, and there have been difficulties matching subjects in control groups (the question of matching for age versus mean length of utterance) (Conti-Ramsden, 1985; Cross, 1984). Another important problem has arisen from the lack of longitudinal studies in this area. Most of the studies have been based on small samples of interaction; for example, Lasky and Klopp (1982) based their study on 15 minutes of analyzed interaction during one session, while Conti-Ramsden and Friel-Patti (1983) considered only 5 minutes from one session.

Despite this controversy, it is important that we not prematurely discard the idea that parental input may influence child language learning. This idea has potential value in the prevention and treatment of language problems. Although there is an absence of conclusive evidence that parental input causes child communication abilities to be either superior or inferior, this absence of evidence cannot be taken as evidence of absence of parental influence (apologies to Carl Sagan). To date, no studies have shown that changing parental input and response *doesn't affect child language behavior.*

Probably the range of possible responses to the child's attempts at communication are similar for both impaired and unimpaired children. What may differ is the frequency with which an impaired child experiences the various responses. If the child's condition or the parents' disposition (influenced by stress, etc.) leads to greater risk of failure to understand or to misinterpretation of the message, the child may experience a higher percentage of negative responses to attempts at communication. Also, if communication attempts are slow, as they often are with the use of augmentative communication devices, interruption is common.

In general, some families, especially those of children with impairments, experience high levels of stress. This stress can easily and frequently cause the family system to become unbalanced. When this occurs, the child's attempts at communcation may meet with less-than-optimal responses.

CONCLUSION

These four important aspects of the impaired child's and his or her family's experience may contribute to delays and failures in the development of communication competence. Consequently, these aspects provide possible targets for prevention and early intervention of communication disorders. Chapter 4 will take a preliminary look at some issues and models of preventive intervention.

Part II

Preventive Intervention in the Family Context

The second section of the book presents a general overview of family-centered intervention, information on the impact of P.L. 99-457, and the skills needed for working with families.

4

Developing a Family-Centered Approach to Preventive Intervention

The first three chapters have provided some information on families and their role in communication development and disorders as background for clinical involvement in family-centered intervention. They have also presented evidence which supports the importance of the family in the treatment process for young children. This kind of evidence has been instrumental in convincing professionals and legislators of the efficacy of family-centered intervention for infants and toddlers.

Unfortunately, knowing why it is important to provide family-centered intervention is only part of the story. We also must know what family-centered services really are and how to develop an approach to services that is truly family centered and that meets the requirements of federal legislation that addresses these services (i.e., P.L. 99-457). In addition, we must become aware of our current practices vis-à-vis families and the attitudes, assumptions, and beliefs that underlie those practices. This awareness is the first step toward changing to a family-centered approach.

In a survey of 67 randomly selected speech-language pathology programs, Crais and Leonard (1990) found that many programs provide limited exposure to areas of information that ". . . have particular relevance for dealing with infants and toddlers who are handicapped and their families and especially for providing interdisciplinary and family-centered services . . ." (pp. 59-60). Similarly, a survey of participants in early intervention-related inservice education programs conducted as part of the Building Blocks project (sponsored by the American Speech-Language-Hearing Association) revealed that only 2 percent of the participants received preservice training that concentrated on infants and toddlers (Catlett, 1991).

This lack of preservice education for participation in family-centered early intervention makes it difficult for administrators to fill the new positions that have been created in response to the new law. Further, when professionals who are already employed in service delivery programs have not developed family-centered attitudes or have difficulty making the ideological "value shift" to family-centered early intervention, it may be because many of its ideas and practices are different from those learned in graduate education.

In addition to the lack of exposure to necessary information, many professionals have been well educated in the traditional model of treatment provision in which professionals make most or all of the decisions about treatment and accept total responsibility for planning and carrying out treatment activities. A closer look at some of the results of traditional early intervention may shed light on the importance of the shift to family-centered services.

TRADITIONAL ASSUMPTIONS AND ATTITUDES IN EARLY INTERVENTION

One of the assumptions that the traditional model of intervention led professionals to make in early intervention was that the clinician could make significant changes in an infant's or toddler's behavior or ability by working with the child alone rather than with the family system. This assumption may create special problems for the family or may lead to lack of lasting progress because the child needs the support of the family in order to make lasting change. Brown (1989) provides a parent's view of this assumption:

> But no matter how we tried as a family to make sense of all the services, of why Aaron was disabled, and of how we would be a family in spite of it, some professional was always there to single out Aaron from the rest of us as needing things that we weren't providing or that they could do better. And there were many professionals to do that! Aaron had a feeding specialist, many physicians in a variety of areas, an OT, a PT and an audiologist as well as the teachers and related staff through the School District. (p. 4)

Efforts at early intervention have often been based on a number of additional assumptions including the notions that: (1) infants are active learners; (2) infant learning can be enhanced by providing certain opportunities and experiences; (3) early experience is important to later development; and (4) early intervention activities are "good for" the child and the family (Healy, Keesee, & Smith, 1985).

Some of these assumptions (i.e., the first and third) have held up well over time, but some should be considered further. For example, the assumption that infant learning can be enhanced with additional experience has sometimes been construed to mean that more opportunities for learning are needed by all at-risk infants. "Infant stimulation" programs have grown from this idea and have provided prescribed stimulation activities for many infants, some of whom were easily overstimulated. The results were often increases in stress that

resulted in infant distress and withdrawal from stimulation rather than prevention of developmental delays.

One important consideration concerning the assumption that early intervention is generally "good for" the child and family is what some people see as the
intrusiveness of early intervention. To be "early," and therefore most effective
and preventive, intervention must occur as soon as a child and family are
suspected of being at-risk or are diagnosed as having an impairment. As
discussed earlier, that time of first learning of the possible problem is a time of
great vulnerability for the family. It is probably a time when the family would
least like to deal with a stranger, no matter how well trained or helpful.
According to Healy et al. (1985):

> Early intervention by its nature is an intimate service that touches a
> family's life at a time of double vulnerability. First, there is the
> normal vulnerability of a family taking on responsibility for a first or
> additional child. Second, there is the often dramatic vulnerability
> brought on by the special-needs situation. These vulnerabilities may
> complicate already existing problems, such as low socioeconomic
> status, unemployment, marital stress or teenaged parenthood. (p. 2)

Without special awareness of families and their needs while adapting to a
child with an impairment or disability, it is easy for professionals, even with the
best of intentions, to increase the stress that family members feel. Awareness of
this special vulnerability may help clinicians to deal more sensitively with
families in need of early intervention services. It will help us to understand the
ambivalence that often greets even our best efforts. Appendix 4-A contains a
parent's reflections on her first experiences with traditional early intervention.
This account makes it clear why some professionals need to reconsider their
interactions with infants and family members.

Another issue that has complicated traditional early intervention efforts is
the history of clinicians' attitudes toward families and their role in communica-
tion/speech-language treatment. Speech-language clinicians have always recognized that parents play an important role in child development. Unfortunately, many professionals were educated during a time when it was popular to
think of parents as contributing to the causes of communication disorders—
genetically (as with Down syndrome), environmentally (e.g., by providing too
little stimulation), or behaviorally (as with Johnson's diagnosogenic model of
stuttering)—but not as contributing in a major way to the planning for or
treatment of communication disorders. We may have emphasized the importance of getting the young child to separate from his mother so that we could
get him into the treatment room without her. We sometimes expected parents to
take responsibility for the most difficult aspect of treatment—carry-over—
without giving them much training to do that. We may have expected parents to

observe us and do what we wrote in the homework notebook. Then we may have been critical and disappointed if they failed to follow through on what seemed to be a clear and reasonable assignment. Other than that, we often didn't expect them to want much more than a five-minute progress report after each treatment session.

Even though we appreciated the importance of parents, some professionals may have had various beliefs and attitudes that made us less-than-optimally helpful to parents. Outspoken parents and professionals have sometimes strongly reminded clinicians of their shortcomings and/or parents' perceptions of professional attitudes (e.g., Darling, 1983; Kupfer, 1984). Vincent (1984) has identified four negative beliefs that professionals have adopted: (1) "parents and family members do not know what their children can do" (p. 37); (2) "parents do not know what appropriate goals are for their children" (p. 38); (3) "[parents] do not know how to teach their kids" (p. 39); and (4) "parents need us" (p. 39).

While these ideas may have some understandable origins, they are certainly not conducive to optimal cooperation between parents and professionals. Further, the first three beliefs listed above have been refuted, for at least some samples of parents, by research (Vincent, 1984). The fourth belief is more difficult. Parents often need the help of professionals and the information that these specialists can provide. Parents don't need experts to come in and take over their rights and responsibilities or to decide what they need to know (Vincent, 1984).

These professional attitudes and practices have been based on a general assumption that the professional should be in control of the treatment situation. That is, that the professional knows best what the client needs and therefore should be the one to decide how to assess communication abilities, plan treatment, and carry out the treatment plan.

In summary, the traditional model of intervention has been one in which clinicians focus on the client's strengths and needs with little or no attention given to the family, and in which they often separate the client from other family members in order to provide assessment and treatment that is planned and carried out by the clinician alone or aided by parents who are given specific assignments. Luterman (1991) has pointed out that this kind of treatment is much like that provided by Annie Sullivan for Helen Keller, and that it allows clinicians to play the role of "rescuers" or "miracle workers." Even though this may be reinforcing and simpler for the clinician, it may not meet the needs of the family or allow for the most effective growth and change of the client.

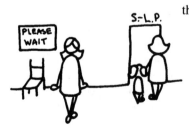

The next section considers a different focus for early intervention efforts—one that puts the family in the forefront of the attempts to provide quality services for infants and toddlers.

FOCUSING ON THE FAMILY

Because of some of our failures and insensitivities, and because of some honest feedback from parents of special needs children, changes have been made in our understanding of families and the role they can and do play in early intervention. To best support the growing child, the family must continue to function as the child's most important developmental context. Family members must continue to play their roles and to maintain that precarious balance as a system. The family's life cycle should proceed as normally as possible. Parents need to be supported in their function as parents, not only as substitute therapists.

In the family-centered model of early intervention, parents, the child's most important advocates, play a very important role in the early intervention process. As Vincent (1984) has stated:

> We're going to need to reorient as professionals. We're going to need to look to parents as leaders, parents as the experts, parents as the bosses. We're going to need to ask them to join us cooperatively as equals in this partnership so that we create a reality out there that matches what all of us want to see. (p. 40)

The family-centered model of intervention differs from the traditional model in that it focuses on the client in the family context, considers the entire family's strengths and needs, and involves family members in assessment, planning of treatment, and in treatment itself at whatever level family members wish to and are capable of being involved. This focus on and involvement of the family is different from the kind of treatment many clinicians were educated to do. It requires that the clinician give up a certain amount of control over the assessment and treatment situation as well as the possibility of feeling like a miracle worker. Instead, the clinician must be able to feel good about helping families to identify and implement what they want for their child and to feel more competent as facilitators of their child's speech and language growth.

Clinicians who make the "value shift" from traditional services and decide that they want to provide family-centered services must gather further information on the nature and methods of family-centered services. For many, this may require a total rethinking of the nature of early intervention.

Perhaps a helpful starting point in thinking about the role clinicians play in family-centered early intervention is with the idea of "intervention" itself. What is intervention? According to the *Merriam-Webster Dictionary* (1974), to intervene is "to come in between in order to stop, settle, or modify" (p. 375). Using this as a starting point, intervention can be seen as an activity that comes between the cause of a problem and the expression of that problem and stops or modifies the outcome. In this sense, intervention can be a preventive activity. Early intervention, then, is an activity or group of activities designed to come between some condition (biological, environmental, etc.) that could cause a problem with development and the expression of that problem at the earliest possible time. The purpose of early intervention is to prevent, or at least lessen, the biological or developmental problems that could result from various risk factors or conditions that predispose a child to a disability or handicap. According to a recent publication of the American Speech-Language-Hearing Foundation (ASHF) (1989):

> Intervention before a problem arises or to keep a problem from getting worse is called *preventive intervention.* Preventive intervention may occur prior to the diagnosis of a delay or disability by reducing exposure for susceptible persons. It may also occur as early detection and treatment of communication disorders which may lead to the elimination of the disorder or the retardation of the disorder's progress, thereby preventing further complications. (p. II-3)

Early or preventive intervention has many different components and can be carried out using many different models of service delivery. These components and models are discussed later in this chapter.

For infants and toddlers, preventive intervention must be carried out within the family context. Intervention that seeks to change only the abilities and behaviors of the infant or toddler overlooks the power of the family system to resist change in one of its members because of the disequilibrium that change may cause, or to facilitate change by adjusting family expectations. It also overlooks the importance of the family environment (the people and the home setting) in the transactional model of development. Only by involving family members in assessment, planning, and intervention can the family system be expected to support and maximize the process of intervention.

Not only are we changing our view of parents and the role that they play in the child's treatment, we are also seeing the importance of other family members in this endeavor. The whole family system, with all of its support potentials and sources of stimulation and interaction, plays a role in the development of the child.

We are also beginning to see this family system in the larger context of its own culture. As clinicians we are recognizing that not all people's values are like our own. Appropriate verbal and nonverbal behavior differs from culture to culture, and our approach to families is beginning to reflect increased sensitivity to these culturally based differences.

A new definition of family-centered care has been developed by the Association for the Care of Children's Health (undated):

Family-centered care is a philosophy of care that recognizes and respects the pivotal role of the family in the lives of children with special health needs. It is a philosophy that strives to support families in their natural caregiving roles by building upon their unique strengths as individuals and as families. It is a philosophy that promotes normal patterns of living at home and in the community. It is a philosophy that views parents and professionals as equals in a partnership committed to excellence at all levels of health care.

This philosophical statement draws together important ideas concerning what families need when they are faced with caring for an infant or toddler who has developmental problems. However, to deliver family-centered services clinicians must go beyond developing or espousing a philosophy. We must take steps to implement the philosophy. Toward that end the National Center for Family-Centered Care (1990) has identified nine key elements of family-centered care.

1. Recognizing that the family is the constant in a child's life, while the service systems and personnel within those systems fluctuate.
2. Facilitating parent/professional collaboration at all levels of health care:
   —care of an individual child
   —program development, implementation, and evaluation
   —policy formation.
3. Honoring the racial, ethnic, cultural, and socioeconomic diversity of families.
4. Recognizing family strengths and individuality and respecting different methods of coping.

5. Sharing with parents, on a continuing basis and in a supportive manner, complete and unbiased information.

6. Encouraging and facilitating family-to-family support and networking.

7. Understanding and incorporating the developmental needs of infants, children, and adolescents and their families into health care systems.

8. Implementing comprehensive policies and programs that provide emotional and financial support to meet the needs of families.

9. Designing accessible health care systems that are flexible, culturally competent, and responsive to family-identified needs.

Operationalizing and applying these key elements to fit into individual service delivery systems is a challenge in which many professionals are currently involved. Crais (1991) suggested that professionals who wish to implement more family-centered practices may find it helpful to use a self-assessment tool such as *Brass Tacks: A Self-Rating of Family-Centered Practices in Early Intervention* (McWilliam & Winton, 1991). (For examples of the items in this rating scale, please see Chapter 10.) McGonigel, Kaufmann, and Johnson (1991) also provide many suggestions for implementing family-centered principles, some of which will be explored later in this text.

FAMILY EMPOWERMENT

As we recognize the importance of the family, we also recognize how easy it is for family members to feel overwhelmed and powerless when a child is identified as having a disabling condition or developmental problem. This often happens because family members can't play their expected roles the way they planned, and because the child cannot play the role the other family members had envisioned for him or her. Suddenly, family members are faced with situations for which they do not have adequate information, and without that information they cannot develop new expectations. They are left with a feeling of frustration and uncertainty in addition to the sense of loss of the "perfect" child. Not only do they not have the dreamed-of child, they aren't able to replace him or her with new expectations. They have lost even their fantasies of what their child will be and how they will be with that child.

This is a time when sensitive professionals can help, not by taking over or by falsely reassuring parents that "everything will be okay", but by facilitating the parents' self-assurance and by giving needed information (Healy et al., 1985).

This has been called "family empowerment," giving, or more accurately, helping the family to gain a feeling of power or competence in the situation (Dunst, Trivette, & Deal, 1988). "A key element in developing appropriate feelings of competence for both the parent and professional is for each to learn when professional expertise is important to decision-making processes, and when the parent is singularly competent to make decisions in the child's best interest" (Healy et al., 1985, p. 38).

One of the major components of the process of empowerment is related to information. Professionals can help family members to feel empowered by giving them, or helping them to gather, needed information. Information, for example, allows them to participate knowledgeably in meetings where decisions concerning their child's treatment will be made, such as the IFSP meeting. In addition, professionals can "enable" family members to feel competent by creating opportunities for competence to be displayed or acquired and by helping them to gain access to and control over the resources that they need (Dunst et al., 1988).

Professionals can also promote family empowerment by helping family members to become appropriately involved in the child's treatment. Parents can be helped to think of themselves not as the source of the child's problems, but as an important part of the treatment effort.

The next section looks at public policy concerning family-centered care and its impact on our practice of early intervention.

EDUCATION OF THE HANDICAPPED ACT AMENDMENTS OF 1986: PUBLIC LAW 99-457, PART H

On October 8, 1986, a new piece of federal legislation was signed into law by President Reagan. This legislation, Public Law (P.L.) 99-457, was designed to amend the original public law concerning education of the handicapped (P.L. 94-142) which was passed in 1975. First, P.L. 99-457 mandates that all state education agencies serve all three-, four-, and five-year-old children by the 1990-1991 school year. In addition, this amendment provides for expanded services to infants and toddlers and their families. It is designed, according to the Administration on Developmental Disabilities (1988), ". . . to support the development of a system within each state that will provide services to very young children with special developmental needs" (p. 9). These services are to be in the form of a "statewide, comprehensive, coordinated, multidisciplinary, interagency program of early intervention services" (P.L. 99-457, 1986, p. 1145).

This portion of the law does not mandate that each state participate in the development of services. It provides for a discretionary program in which states may choose to participate. However, after four years, states that wish to continue receiving federal funds for programs that serve the birth through two- and three- to five-year-old populations must have programs to provide appropriate early intervention to all handicapped infants and toddlers in the state.

Although there are four parts to this legislation, it is Title I that is of greatest importance for family-centered early intervention. This section of the act outlines the purpose and requirements of the birth through two programs that are to be funded under this law. As stated in the law, the purposes of the programs for infants and toddlers are:

> . . . to enhance the development of handicapped infants and toddlers and minimize their potential for developmental delay; reduce the education costs to our society, including our schools; . . . minimize the likelihood of institutionalization; . . . and enhance the capacity of families to meet the special needs of their infants and toddlers with handicaps. (p. 1145)

The law states that infants and toddlers are eligible for these programs if they

1. are experiencing developmental delays as measured by appropriate diagnostic instruments and procedures in one or more of the following areas: cognitive development, physical development, language and speech development, psychosocial development, or self-help skills, or
2. have a diagnosed physical or mental condition which has a high probability of resulting in developmental delay. (p. 1146)

States may also include, at their own discretion, infants and toddlers who are "at risk of having substantial developmental delays if early intervention services are not provided" (p. 1146).

The services to be provided for infants and toddlers and their families are defined as follows:

> Early intervention services are developmental services which—
> • are provided under public supervision
> • are provided at no cost except where federal or state law provides for a system of payments by families including a schedule of sliding fees
> • are designed to meet a handicapped infant's or toddler's developmental needs in any one or more of the following areas:

—physical development
—cognitive development
—language and speech development
—psychosocial development or self-help skills
- meet the standards of the state, including the requirements of this part, including
  —family training, counseling, and home visits
  —special instruction
  —speech pathology and audiology
  —occupational therapy
  —physical therapy
  —psychological services
  —case management services
  —medical services only for diagnostic or evaluation purposes
  —early identification, screening, and assessment services
  —health services necessary to enable the infant or toddler to benefit from the other early intervention services
- are provided by qualified personnel, including
  —special educators
  —speech and language pathologists and audiologists
  —occupational therapists
  —physical therapists
  —psychologists
  —social workers
  —nurses
  —nutritionists
- are provided in conformity with an individualized family service plan adopted in accordance with section 677. (pp. 1146-1147)

The statewide system must include at least the following components:

- a definition of the term *developmentally delayed*
- time tables for ensuring full services to all eligible children
- multidisciplinary evaluations of each child and of the needs of their families
- Individualized Family Service Plans (IFSP)
- a public awareness program
- a central directory of services, experts, etc.

- a comprehensive system of personnel development
- a Lead Agency designated by the governor which oversees the statewide system
- a policy for contracting with service providers
- a procedure for securing reimbursement of funds from other agencies responsible for services
- procedural safeguards
- professional standards (adapted from "Fact Sheet P.L. 99-457")

The provisions of this law appear to have taken into account many important aspects of the delivery of services to infants and toddlers and their families. In the reauthorization of this act the 101st Congress changed the name of the Education of the Handicapped Act to Individuals with Disabilities Education Act (IDEA) and changed the terminology of the law. For example, the term *handicap* was replaced with *disability* and *handicapped infants and toddlers* became *infants and toddlers with disabilities* (McGonigel et al., 1991). The requirements of the law will be discussed further in other sections of this book.

The following section considers different models of intervention which can be used to implement family-centered services such as those called for by P.L. 99-457.

EARLY INTERVENTION MODELS

Once the decision has been made to provide family-centered services, there are a number of alternative models of intervention to choose from. The major choices for services include: (1) the composition of the multidisciplinary intervention team and the degree of service coordination; (2) the context in which services will be delivered; (3) the expected outcome of services; and (4) the components of treatment to be offered. Each of these aspects of early intervention service delivery will be discussed below.

Team Composition and Service Coordination

Even before the passage of P.L. 94-142 it was clear that intervention with very young children who had multiple developmental and health problems required a team of professionals who were able to supply the different pieces of information needed to solve treatment problems. The membership of the multidisciplinary team that is required for any given child and family depends on the individual needs of that child and family. Any or all of the following people may be members of a team: family members, speech-language pathologists, audiologists, special educators, occupational therapists, physical therapists, nurses, physicians, nutritionists, dentists or orthodontists, and psychologists.

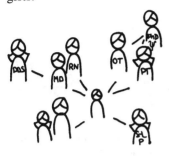

The members of the team may play a number of different roles depending on the model of service delivery adopted and the needs of the family. Team members may provide direct service in the form of support or treatment specific to their specialty. They may provide consultation in which they share their expertise with other team members, including family members, so that those members can deliver more comprehensive direct service. Team members may act as educators, teaching other professionals, family members, or the general public about their field. Or they may take the role of care coordinator or case manager (sometimes called "service coordinator"). The care coordinator (1) schedules and coordinates assessment from all team members, (2) provides leadership in the development of the IFSP, (3) assists the family to identify service providers and support organizations in the community, and (4) coordinates, monitors, and ensures timely delivery of early intervention services (ASHA, 1989).

There are four possible levels of service coordination which may be used when professionals from different fields are involved with a family: (1) independent, (2)

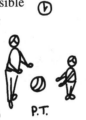

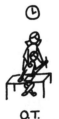

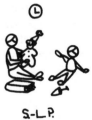

P.T.   O.T.   S-L.P.

multidisciplinary, (3) interdisciplinary, and (4) transdisciplinary. With *independent* services each professional works independently with no plan for collaboration. There is no sense of the professional as a member of a team.

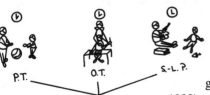

P.T.   O.T.   S-L.P.

The term *multidisciplinary* has been used in two different ways. It has been used as a generic term for coordinated services which have some formal mechanism for sharing information in general (McCormick & Schiefelbusch, 1990), and as a specific term to denote a team approach in which professionals play their own, traditional roles with little, if any, coordination of services (McCormick & Schiefelbusch, 1990; Wilcox, 1989).

In what has been called the *interdisciplinary* model, various professionals work together on the evaluation and treatment team, but each separately evaluates and treats the child and family, maintaining his or her traditional professional role. The interdisciplinary team establishes formal channels for communication and collaboration, and a case manager or care coordinator is often assigned to coordinate services (McCormick & Schiefelbusch, 1990).

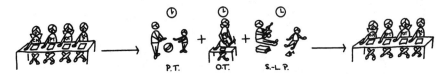

The *transdisciplinary* model is characterized by the greatest degree of coordination of any of the team models. In this approach, professionals share their expertise with one another, cooperating to the degree that several team members may provide only indirect service to a child and family while other members do all of the hands-on assessment and intervention. Lyon and Lyon (1980) have identified joint functioning (team members work together when possible), continuous staff development (members train one another), and role release (members may give up their direct service roles and provide consultation to another member who provides the service) as three characteristics of the transdisciplinary model. One unique practice of some transdisciplinary teams is "arena assessment" in which participating team members, including the parents, watch as a single "assessment facilitator" works with the child. Team members may ask that certain test items be administered as they watch, and they can observe the child in interaction without the stress for the child of being handled or asked to perform by many people (McCormick & Schiefelbusch, 1990).

Of these different models of service coordination, the transdisciplinary model is perhaps the most suited to family-centered early intervention. As active members of the assessment and treatment team some family members may be willing and able to take the role of the hands-on, primary therapist with other team members providing expertise through a consultation model. The very young child, therefore, interacts primarily with his or her parent or other family member and may receive facilitative interaction continuously, rather than only when taken to special treatment sessions. When this is not desirable or possible, this approach is still an especially good one for infants and toddlers and their families because they deal directly with fewer professionals and the care is less difficult to coordinate and schedule.

While the team approach is both desired and required in early intervention, developing a working team of professionals is not simply accomplished by locating and contracting with individuals who have the necessary expertise. Briggs (1991) has emphasized the importance of preparing individual team members for participation on a team and of developing a team decision-making process. She has also stressed that teams typically go through several stages of development before they become productive and function well together.

Context and Nature of Services

A second consideration in selecting an early intervention model is the context in which services should be delivered and the basic nature of those services. The context or location of service delivery can either be center/school-based or home-based.

Center/School-Based Services

Center/school-based services are provided in an institutional setting, perhaps a private agency, a hospital, or local education agency, often with the child participating with other children in group experiences of some kind. Unless 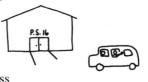 the child is living in the center or school, as he or she might be in a hospital neonatal or pediatric intensive care unit (NICU or PICU), services that are delivered away from home require that the child be transported to the service delivery site. Most center/school-based programs emphasize direct work of professionals with the child, although there is an attempt to involve the parents or other family members at some level.

Home-Based Treatment

Home-based treatment, of course, takes place in the child's home and requires that professional(s) travel to that location. Home-based treatment is often designed to teach parents to work with their infants and toddlers, and consequently requires a higher level of parent/family involvement than most center/school-based programs. The "pay-off" of this high level of family involvement is often that the child receives much more concentrated treatment—treatment that can, in the case of therapeutic language input, be carried out during most of his or her waking hours. Other benefits of home-based treatment include the decreased cost of services (Barnett & Escobar, 1989; Shearer & Shearer, 1976), and the fact that in the home all important aspects of the child's "ecosystem" (Bricker & Carlson, 1981) can be included in treatment.

Shearer and Shearer (1976) list seven educational advantages of home-based programs.

1. Learning occurs in the parent and child's natural environment; therefore, the typical problem of transferring back into the home what has been learned in a classroom or clinic does not exist.

2. There is direct and constant access to behavior as it occurs naturally . . . [and] the differences in cultures, life styles, and value systems held by the parents are incorporated into curriculum planning.

3. It is more likely that learned behavior will generalize and be maintained.

4. There is more opportunity for full family participation in the teaching process.

5. There is access to the full range of behaviors.

6. It is hypothesized that the training of parents, who already are natural reinforcing agents, will provide them with the skills necessary to deal with new behaviors when they occur.

7. Finally, because the home teacher is working on a one-to-one basis with the parents and child, individualization of instructional goals for both is an operational reality. (pp. 336-337)

Integrated vs. Segregated Settings

A second parameter of the context in which services are delivered is the issue of whether center/school-based services are delivered in an integrated (participating children may be normally developing or impaired/at risk) or a segregated (participating children all have impairments or risk factors) setting. This is not a major issue for most public facilities because few states provide preschool services for children who do not have disabilities. It has been an issue for older Head Start children because legislation mandates that a percentage of children in these programs be "handicapped."

And it is a concern for some private facilities who serve both normally developing children and children with disabilities.

Integration of services has often been promoted with the intent of facilitating peer interactions and providing a model of normal child behavior for children with developmental problems (Campbell, 1989b). Unfortunately, just putting normally developing children with children with disabilities in the same facility does not necessarily promote interaction. Activities must be specifically designed to promote sustained and communicative interactions. Under such conditions, language-impaired children do seem to communicate more readily when grouped with normal language users (McCormick & Schiefelbusch, 1990).

The issue of facilitating peer interactions is of much greater concern for children more than three years of age than it is for infants and toddlers. For children less than three, family interactions are of greater importance. Home-based services allow for inclusion of older siblings in language-promoting interactions. Incorporating siblings into the language treatment program may serve the same goals as do integrated treatment settings.

Clinician/Trainer-Oriented vs. Child-Oriented Treatment

The basic nature of the treatment that will be provided is a final consideration for preventive intervention. Programs in which the clinician selects the goals, stimuli, procedures, correct responses, and reinforcement to be used are clinician/trainer-oriented programs. The trainer is, or attempts to be, in control of the language learning situation (Fey, 1986). These programs are usually based on operant learning theory and have their origins in behavioral therapy. They are usually conducted under controlled conditions, as in a clinical setting, rather than in natural settings. The interactions that take place in this kind of treatment are not those typical of normal communicative interaction.

Child-oriented treatment is quite different from clinician/trainer-oriented treatment. In child-oriented treatment the clinician attempts to create an atmosphere and environment that will facilitate and encourage the child's spontaneous communication. Rather than deciding upon the stimuli, procedures, and other input that the child must respond to, the clinician follows the child's lead in attention, play, and conversation and responds using various language facilitating techniques such as expansions and expatiations (Fey, 1986). Child-oriented treatment has been referred to using terms such as *incidental language teaching* and *natural language treatment.*

Child-oriented treatment is especially suited to family-centered, home-based treatment. Once parents and other family members learn the language facilitation techniques they can provide natural and on-going language treatment while carrying on with their daily routines.

Expected Outcomes of Treatment

We would like to think of early intervention as always eradicating the threatened language or speech problem. Unfortunately, the outcome of our efforts is not always complete prevention of communication disorders. Realistically, we may expect the outcome of intervention to be one of three conditions: prevention, remediation, or compensation (ASHA, 1989). When intervention is implemented before any symptoms of disordered communication occur and such symptoms are inhibited from occurring, prevention has taken place. This outcome can also be called primary prevention (ASHA, 1988).

After symptoms of a communication disorder have been identified and diagnosed, we often engage in efforts to improve function and eliminate as many of the symptoms as possible. In this case, the efforts result in remediation of the problem (ASHA, 1989).

When conditions that put a child at risk for a communication disorder are unalterable (as, for example, with severe oral motor problems), there may be no way to prevent or eliminate the symptoms of disordered communication. When this is true our efforts to decrease the effects of this condition by helping the child to learn and to use alternative strategies or augmentative techniques result in compensation.

All three of these outcomes may be the focus of early intervention for different children or for different aspects of one child's problem. The goal is always to enhance functional communication ability.

Components of Intervention

Early intervention programs must provide five components of intervention: (1) screening/identification, (2) assessment/observation, (3) treatment/support, (4) ongoing evaluation, and (5) care coordination. These components of intervention may be provided using any of the models of service delivery discussed above.

Screening or identification of young children who are at risk for communication disorders is not a simple process. The intent is to select those children who should be further assessed for signs of communication deficit or for conditions that may lead to such a problem. When there is an obvious medical or genetic condition, such as premature birth or Down syndrome, this identification may take place at or shortly after birth. With less obvious conditions, such as hearing loss, it may take much longer and may rely upon parental observation and knowledge of normal behavior and development. "Child find" efforts are now being instituted to increase the percentage of babies who are identified early in life.

The second step in early intervention is assessment and observation of the child and family. In family-centered early intervention the family's strengths and needs are also to be identified as part of the assessment process. One of our most important roles in assessment of the family may be consideration of the family as a context for language learning. Assessment of the infant's or toddler's abilities as a communicator is a challenge. It requires a strong grounding in normal infant and toddler development with special emphasis on prelinguistic and early verbal communication. It also requires excellent observation skills which can be used to gather information on parent-child communicative interaction. In addition, skill in administering formal assessment tools as well as informal probes, often under less-than-optimal conditions, is required.

The first step in providing treatment and support for very young children and their families is planning the intervention in collaboration with the family. P.L. 99-457 requires the development of an IFSP which specifies the goals and procedures to be implemented. After a treatment plan is agreed upon, intervention is provided following the plan with special attention to giving support to family members. Treatment progress must be evaluated on a regular basis to be sure that the planned intervention is having the expected success.

Because many young children who need early intervention services require several kinds of treatment, care coordination is a necessary component of most programs. (See section on "Team Composition" for a discussion of care coordination or case management.)

CONCLUSION

These different models of early intervention are practiced in various intervention settings. While P.L. 99-457 calls for certain common components in all programs, there is still some room for flexibility in program development and each family requires an individualized combination of services.

Chapter 5 will consider some of the special skills that professionals need for working with families.

Appendix 4-A

One Parent's Reaction to Traditional Early Intervention

The day I found the early intervention center, I cried with relief. It seemed like the answer to our prayers: on-staff physical therapist, speech therapist, occupational therapist, instructor and social worker. The program was free to all who had at-risk babies and only six blocks from our apartment. Our baby son Jesse was certainly at risk: he was nine weeks premature and had suffered a Grade IV intraventricular hemorrhage. He has been diagnosed with mild to moderate cerebral palsy, and we wanted to begin a comprehensive program for him as soon as possible. When we started at the early intervention center, Jesse was seven months old—five and a half months old when corrected for prematurity.

The room where the program took place was cavernous, with high ceilings lit by florescent lights and a sound quality that both raised and muffled normal speech tones. On our first day, Jesse was strapped into a reclined seater and placed in a semicircle with the other infants, parents seated behind and the instructor in the middle. The instructor began singing a song naming the infants and parents, then took the babies through a sequence of banging on a drum, shaking rattles and ringing bells. Jesse reacted badly to the lights, noise and restraints and began screaming and thrashing in his chair. The instructor addressed him firmly, saying: "Jesse. When you stop crying, you can come out of the chair." Jesse somehow ignored this helpful advice, his screams accelerating to an hysterical pitch. I was told that all the babies reacted this way at first, and that Jesse would get used to it. I was not allowed to take him out of the chair and comfort him because "CP kids have to learn independence." Finally, Jesse shut everyone out, gazing fixedly to the side. I was told that this classic display of preemie avoidance "could be a seizure."

That night, I paced the floor, smoking, crying and feeling helpless. For the first time I felt that we had a handicapped child, not a baby who might possibly

Source: From "Early Intervention or Early Interference? One Family's Experience" by M. Leone, 1989, *The Networker, 2,* pp. 5, 20. Copyright 1989 by United Cerebral Palsy Associations, Inc.

have a handicap. But every book I had read, every professional we had consulted had all stressed the need for early intervention. Our baby who had not been "our" baby for the seven weeks he was in the hospital neonatal intensive care unit was *still* not our baby. We were told how to hold, bathe and feed him, information we needed but still resented. When my husband had casually mentioned that we took our baby into our bed at night, a horrified chorus of voices at the center reacted as if we were performing sex acts on our child. "You'll put a strain on your marriage!" cried those young, single, childless women. How could they know the feelings of love and closeness we experienced as we cuddled our baby? Their advice was an intrusion. It had nothing to do with cerebral palsy, and I showed my resentment by stubbornly refusing to listen to them.

Our session with the physical therapist was also a disaster. As she roughly stripped Jesse of his outside clothes, he began to howl. "Well, I can't work with him if he's going to cry all the time. Won't he take a pacifier?" No, he wouldn't—maybe because of the tongue-thrusting that I had seen no evidence of but that the speech therapist insisted he must have. The speech therapist also informed me that although he was age-appropriate for language, he would definitely have problems pronouncing his d's, b's, and p's; all CP children did. I worried about his future speech problems, thinking sadly that even his small triumphs were short-lived. A week and a half later, he began saying, "dih-gee."

Things improved somewhat when I asked the instructors to dim the lights during the sessions. I also requested that Jesse be allowed to come out of the chair at the first signs of hysteria. I would then calm him down and try to return him to the chair in a little while. The instructors agreed, but the next hurdle I faced was the inflexibility of scheduling, even when it bordered on the absurd. During one session I was informed that it was the day for "parent group" and I should leave Jesse with the instructors and attend. Noting that the only other parents present were two other mothers who didn't speak English, I politely declined, suggesting we use the time to work with Jesse. No, today was the day for parent's group. So I spent forty-five minutes listening to the social worker explain in fractured Spanish how to get social service benefits to the two women who sat nodding and smiling to my right and left. Through it all, I could hear Jesse screaming in the next room. Released from this fiasco, I arrived back just in time to hear the speech therapist telling my son, "Jesse. When you stop crying, you can. . . ." I interrupted her by reaching over, unstrapping my son and taking him in my arms. She glared at me and said, "You'd better start feeding him in a seat. Otherwise, he's going to look like *this*." And she mimed a severely spastic, rigid child.

The next morning I found myself wrestling anxiously with Jesse during breakfast, the image of the rigid child before my eyes like a nightmare vision of the future. He cried, I cried, and no breakfast was eaten that day.

The uneaten meal marked the turning point. I cancelled the appointment with the physical therapist at the center and hired a gentle, positive therapist who made home visits. She didn't even touch Jesse until near the end of the first session, and he is now making consistent progress. We withdrew Jesse from the program and bought lots of books. My husband and I knew the neuro-developmental techniques for holding, feeding and bathing our child, and Jesse doesn't miss the "stimulation" of being restrained in a chair and having bells and rattles shaken at him. He is registered in a new program in another town, one my husband and I learned about from a program on public broadcasting. But at the first signs of negativity, insensitivity, bullying or ignorance, we will withdraw from this program, too.

Professionals need to realize the damage that harsh lights and jangling sounds can do to the baby with an immature central nervous system. Parents should become actively involved with their child's stimulation and therapy. The way to encourage that involvement is to empower the parents and impress upon them the need to carry over handling and feeding techniques into the daily routine. Worst-case scenarios and dire predictions foster a sense of helplessness compounded by anxiety and depression. The parent of an at-risk child is in a situation where many different types of professionals are all giving assorted, often conflicting advice on every aspect of raising that child. If the parent makes a personal choice on an aspect of child care that has nothing to do with that child's health problem, let the parents assume control in that area. Try not to regard or refer to the child as his or her disability. To the parent, that child is a unique individual, and the professionals should be able to see the child, not the handicap. If this is not possible, that professional does not belong in the health care profession.

Our baby is a miracle of survival. We are thrilled by his progress and will not allow limitations to be placed on him. Nothing less than his future is at stake.

In addition to being the proud parents of 15-month-old Jesse, Marianne Leone and her husband, Chris Cooper, are also professional actors. Marianne appears in "True Love," a film that will be released next fall, and Chris was recently seen in the role of July Johnson in the TV mini-series, "Lonesome Dove."

5

Special Skills for Working with Families

Family-centered intervention requires some special skills or adaptations of existing skills. This chapter will consider family-centered applications of clinical interviewing, counseling, and consultation.

CLINICAL INTERVIEWING

Clinical interviewing is a special kind of language used by many human service professionals both as a tool to gather information and as a support-giving skill which is part of our counseling techniques. Patton (1980) stated that the purpose of interviewing is "to allow us to enter into the other person's perspective" (p. 196). He outlined three approaches to collecting qualitative information through interviewing: (1) informal conversational interviewing; (2) the general interview guide approach; and (3) the standardized open-ended interview. These approaches differ in the level of preplanning of questions that is involved. For the informal conversational interview there is little, if any, preplanning. The interviewer relies on spontaneous questions that occur in the course of an interaction with the interviewee. According to Patton, this approach is most useful when there's no presupposition on the part of the interviewer about what information might be important. This kind of interview allows the interviewer to follow the interviewee's lead, but it relies heavily on the interviewer's skill and takes more time and effort to collect systematic information and to analyze data (Patton, 1980).

The general interview guide approach involves more preplanning of the questions to be asked. The interviewer begins with an outline of issues to be explored, but without standardized questions. This helps to focus the interview and can make interviewing systematic and comprehensive when more than one person is to be querried (Patton, 1980).

With the standardized open-ended interview, exact questions to be asked, and often the sequence in which they are asked, are specified. This level of preplanning often saves time, improves reliability when interview results are to be compared, and makes data analysis easier (Patton, 1980).

The fourth approach to interviewing, closed quantitative interviewing, specifies both the interviewer's questions and the interviewee's possible responses (Patton, 1980). This type of questionnaire interviewing greatly restricts and may distort the information obtained in the interview (Patton, 1980).

When clinicians use interviews to gather information, we most often use a general interview guide approach with a loosely specified outline of topics to be explored. Clinical interviewing as a support-giving skill will most often employ the informal conversational approach so that the interviewer can readily respond to the concerns of the interviewee.

Many sources supply information on the basics of interviewing as a clinical skill. For example, Cormier and Cormier (1985), Garrett (1970), Ivey (1971), and Winton (1988) all presented lists of interviewing behaviors that can be mastered. Drawing upon these sources we can compile an annotated list of interviewing skills.

Background Skills	
Observation	gathering information by watching client behaviors
Attending behavior	nonverbal and verbal behavior that shows the client that you are interested in him or her (e.g., relaxed, natural posture; comfortable eye contact; comments which relate to the interviewee's statements [Ivey, 1971])
Invitations to Talk	
Open questions	questions that allow the respondent to talk at length on a topic that is only broadly specified by the interviewer (Cormier & Cormier, 1985; Ivey, 1971) (e.g., "Could you tell me how your baby communicates with you?")
Closed questions	questions which specify the information that is to be given. Closed questions can often be answered in a few words (Cormier & Cormier, 1985; Ivey, 1971). (e.g., "Does your baby point to things he or she wants?")
Minimal encouragements	interviewer responses designed to keep the interviewee talking (e.g., "m-m-h-m-m," "Oh?," "Tell me more," head nodding, expectant eye contact)
Listening Skills	
Reflection of feeling	interviewer responses that focus on and label the feelings or affect expressed by the interviewee (Cormier & Cormier, 1985; Ivey, 1971) (e.g., "You

	feel pretty angry about your treatment by the people at that clinic.")
Paraphrase of content	interviewer responses that focus on and rephrase the content of the interviewee's message (Cormier & Cormier, 1985; Ivey, 1971) (e.g., "The doctors and nurses asked a lot of questions that seemed irrelevant to you.")
Summarization	interviewer statements that recapitulate, condense, or clarify the interviewee's feelings and/or content in the whole session or a major portion thereof (Cormier & Cormier, 1985; Ivey, 1971) (e.g., "For the last few months you've been trying to find appropriate services for your child, but it's been difficult, and you've often felt frustrated. You've almost given up hope.")
Expressive Responses	
Responses to personal questions	interviewer responses to client's direct questions about himself or herself. Garrett (1970) suggests that answers be brief and followed by a redirection (e.g., "I'm from northern New England. Let's talk now about the problem you mentioned with feeding.")
Expression of feeling/ content	interviewer's verbalization of his or her own feelings, thoughts, etc. (e.g., "When my son was tiny I often had questions about how to care for him. I felt a lot of confusion.")
Confrontation	the interviewer notes and describes a discrepancy in the interviewee's behaviors (e.g., "You have said that you would like to work on ____, but each time we begin to do so you bring up some other issue.")
Interpretation	an interviewer comment on interviewee content and/ or feelings which goes beyond what the interviewee has expressed by noting an association between behaviors or events or attempting to explain behaviors (Cormier & Cormier, 1985; Ivey, 1971) (e.g., "It seems as though you're afraid that your new baby may have some of the problems that ____ has.")
Information giving	the interviewer verbally communicates facts (e.g., "Our center-based program meets from 10:00 to 1:00 on Monday, Wednesday, and Friday.")

Because questions are so frequently used in interviewing, they may deserve a bit of extra attention. Patton (1980) has identified six kinds of questions: (1) experience/behavior questions that request descriptions of behaviors; (2) opinion/

value questions that seek information on beliefs; (3) feeling questions that try to gather information on emotions; (4) knowledge questions that solicit responses concerning factual information; (5) sensory questions that request information on what is seen, heard, etc.; and (6) background/demographic questions that gather identifying information about the respondent. Patton (1980) stresses that the best questions are singular (only one question is asked at a time) and clearly stated in the same terms used by the respondent and without unfamiliar jargon.

One efficient way to master these techniques is to use a microtraining approach (Ivey, 1971). As practiced by Ivey, this technique employs a systematic approach to learning. Each component skill of interviewing is learned separately following a progression: (1) a trainee completes a videotaped interview with a volunteer client; (2) the client evaluates the session; (3) the trainee reads material describing an interview skill that he or she then discusses with a supervisor; (4) the trainee views video models of the technique; (5) the trainee is shown and discusses with the supervisor his or her initial interview, identifying instances where he or she used or failed to use the interview skill; (6) the supervisor and trainee review the skill; and (7) the trainee reinterviews the same client attempting to use the skill more effectively and receives feedback and evaluation. Each skill is practiced separately and then added to skills previously mastered (Ivey, 1971).

These skills are usually taught with a great deal of emphasis on the interviewer behaviors to be used and less attention to the possible interviewee responses. There often seems to be emphasis on using these verbal tools to help the interviewee "open up" while guarding the interviewer's personal anonymity and privacy. For example, Garrett (1970) states,

> Sometimes an interviewer deliberately introduces his own personal interests into the discussion. . . . Although at times such devices may be successful in helping the interviewee to feel acquainted and relaxed, the value of their use except in rare instances is dubious. Their dangers outweigh their possible value. (p. 42)

A less formal approach to managing verbal interactions may be useful in some clinical situations. Both Goodman and Esterly (1988) and Miller, Wackman,

Nunnally, and Saline (1982) have written about the use of communication in human interaction. Their information and suggestions for enhancing communication appear to be adaptations of more formal interviewing skills and may be useful techniques for both clinicians and clients to learn and use. (The issue of using less formal communication skills will be discussed below.) Goodman and Esterly (1988), for example, present the following list of "talk tools."

Disclosures	". . . simple revelations of personal history" (p. 3).
	For example: (Parent) "I've found it really hard to tell my parents about the baby's problem. I still haven't told them that he'll need several operations. They think he'll be OK after this first time in the hospital."
	(Clinician) "Before I had children I didn't understand why parents had such a hard time disciplining their children. I thought it was a pretty simple procedure. Now that I'm dealing with it with my own children, I see some of the things that make it so difficult."
Reflections	Statements that "show that meaning has registered . . . [and] tell the listener that he or she has been *heard*" (p. 38 emphasis in original).
	For example: (Clinician) "You feel as though you understand all of the reasons that Timmy is having a hard time staying with a play activity, but you still find it frustrating."
	(Parent to parent) "It sounds as if you're having just as hard a time accepting this problem as I am."
Advisements	Statements designed to provide guidance in the form of "advising questions" ("Why don't you . . ."), "me too advisements" ("I know what you mean, my _____ does ___, too, but I . . ."), suggestions, and commands.
	For example: (Clinician) "Several mothers have told me that they had a similar problem with slowing their speech down when they talked to their toddler. They found that it was easier to start slowing down when they read a story to their child. Perhaps you could try that."
Interpretations	Statements that offer new meaning, generalizations about human nature, or insights into personality.
	For example: (Parent to parent) "I've heard you say that same thing in every meeting we've had, that you're not worried about the way Johnny repeats things. Since you keep thinking and talking about it, I wonder if you really are worried."
Questions	Often meant to gather information but may also be used to advise, interpret, or disclose.

	For example: "Can you try ignoring the behavior?" (advisement); "Do you think he might want you to let him try it himself?" (interpretation); "Can you imagine how dumb I felt?" (disclosure).
Silences	Pauses in conversation that "regulate the flow of listening and talking" (p. 147).
	For example: (Parent) "So I guess I'll try to be more patient." (Clinician is silent, but looks at the parent expectantly.) "I mean, I won't just do it for him, I'll wait and see if he can work it out himself."

These skills, while similar, and in some cases identical, to the interviewing skills discussed earlier, emphasize both "client/interviewee" and "clinician/interviewer" communication behavior. Goodman and Esterly's (1988) discussion of the skills stresses the complementary use of behaviors by both parties.

Using Clinical Interviewing Skills in Family-Centered Early Intervention

The idea of family members as full-fledged team members working in an "equal partnership" with professionals, which was discussed in Chapter 4, has important implications for our use of clinical interviewing behaviors. The professional interviewing behaviors which we have adopted and developed over the years are designed to maintain the separate and unequal roles of clinician/interviewer and client/interviewee. They promote a kind of communication that requires self-disclosure from the interviewee but forbids such disclosure from the interviewer. This behavior has worked well to keep the sometimes-desired distance between professionals and patients. In fact, we have taught and practiced these skills with emphasis on the importance of maintaining this difference and never allowing a lapse into the two-sided give and take of "conversation."

It may be that we cannot have an "equal partnership" or function as co-workers with family members as long as we use our traditional interviewing skills in a formal manner. If we do use formal skills, the result may be a one-sided relationship in which the family member discloses private or painful information and the professional responds in a nonpersonal, nonequal manner. As Goodman and Esterly (1988) point out,

> In nonprofessional close relationships, when only one person is vulnerable to the other over an extended period, the relationship loses its balance of power, its equality of access. The symmetry that gives intimacy its start must extend into the giving and taking of openness. If not, the human connection becomes unstable. (pp. 186-187)

Even though our intent is not to build intimate relationships with our client/co-workers, if we are to function as true equals, we may need to modify our expectations and behaviors in the interviewing situation.

In addition to this issue of team member equality, there is a question of the validity of information gained from the use of formal interviewing skills. Briggs (1986) points out that a certain kind of "communication event" (p. 2) takes place when one person is interviewed by another. Participation in this communication event requires that both parties abide by certain communication rules and play certain roles which are not necessarily in concert with the rules and roles they normally use or play. So, in an interview we, to some extent, put aside who we really are and how we usually talk, and we participate in an interaction which is a rather formal event, designed especially to exchange information. While this situation may be an efficient way to gather information, it may bias the quality and/or quantity of information gained. According to Briggs (1986), "The social situation created by the interview does not simply constitute an obstacle to the respondents' articulation of his or her beliefs. Like speech events in general, it shapes the form and content of what is said" (p. 22).

In addition, Briggs (1986) suggests that the interviewee may come from a community whose sociolinguistic norms are very different from those of the interview situation or the interviewer. This issue is of special importance when working with families from other cultures or when interviewees come from groups that do not usually participate in interviews and may therefore be unwilling or unable to abide by its rules. In some cases, a culture's communication rules may directly prohibit the respondent from giving the information that the interviewer seeks. And in some families, certain topics simply aren't discussed. For example, an interviewer's attempts to uncover information about the support available to a mother may be frustrated by the unwritten rule "never complain about family to a stranger."

In summary, the "product" or information that results from an interview is usually considered true information about the interviewee or the family. We usually have little awareness that this information is a product of an unusual interaction which was obtained under very special circumstances. These circumstances may have negatively influenced the interview's validity (Briggs, 1986).

Another issue that impacts on our use of interviewing skills in family-centered intervention is our actual mastery of the skills. As professionals who are especially concerned about enhancing communication, speech-language pathologists seem to be in a perfect position to excell at interviewing. Unfortunately, this complex skill is sometimes taught to student clinicians in a cursory manner or by people who know little about it themselves. We may begin our work with clients with inadequate confidence in our ability to interview and with little actual skill to share. Even when our skills are solid and well rehearsed, we may be ill prepared to respond to the information that the skills elicit from clients. In fact, we may seldom have considered the communication skills the client may use in response to our interviewing behaviors.

In addition, Winton and Bailey (1990) have pointed out that interviewing skills designed for use in individual sessions may not be adequate for interviews with groups such as families. We may need special skills such as encouraging equal participation and managing conflict in order to work well with families. Unfortunately, it is difficult to learn interviewing skills, especially those skills needed to work with family groups, from articles and texts. The best way to master these skills is through well-supervised practicum experience and repeated trial and error. (In fact, "errors" may be necessary to the learning process.) Videotaping, analyzing, and critiquing your interviewing skills, especially with the help and support of a knowledgeable supervisor, may hasten the process of mastery.

In summary, our clinical interviewing skills may need to be adapted to the special demands of family-centered early intervention. Although we still need to use our communication skills consciously and carefully when we communicate with family members who are equals on the intervention team, we may want to downplay some of the external trappings of the interviewer role. It may be especially helpful to engage in some cautious and well-considered self-disclosure.

Adapting Interviewing Skills

Perhaps the best preparation for this adapted form of clinical interviewing is to study and master both traditional interviewing skills and the more informal "talk tools" as presented by Goodman and Esterly (1988). When working with families, the first interview-related goal might be to gain an understanding of the communicative norms of the family's culture (Briggs, 1986). Briggs suggests a number of ways to increase the value of the interview information such as becoming acquainted with the community in which the family lives, learning the language or dialect, observing who talks to whom, who listens to whom, when people talk, how people ask questions, and who can ask questions of whom. In other words, he suggests learning about the context in which communication takes place and discovering the ways in which people communicate both verbally and nonverbally. We can begin to do this by spending time with the family and observing their interactions to gain information that will supplement the interview data.

If we are going to be using interviewing skills or talk tools, we can help family members to learn to use these tools as well. This information will not only increase their ability to communicate interpersonally and to provide a useful language model for their child, it will also allow them to participate as equals with us in information exchange situations. Chapter 6 contains further information on the use of interviewing skills in family assessment.

EXERCISE #1

If you are not a practiced and confident clinical interviewer, find a group of people with whom you can practice interviewing. Set up role playing situations or interview each other about actual life events. Videotape your interviews and critique your own performance. Role play a family interview to get a feel for the difference in group dynamics.

COUNSELING AND FAMILY THERAPY TECHNIQUES

Clinicians' work with families often presents opportunities for the use of counseling skills. The ability to enter into a counseling relationship with family members goes well beyond our use of interviewing skills. Both education and the creation of a growth-enhancing relationship are important components of its definition. Counseling, as defined by Luterman (1984), is ". . . an educative experience occurring between people, which is problem-centered and allows for the expression of feeling (affect), permitting and encouraging growth in both parties" (p. 2).

Focusing specifically on counseling parents of children with special needs, Stewart (1986) states,

> Counseling is a helping relationship between a knowledgeable professional and the parents [or other family members] of an exceptional child who are working toward a better understanding of their unique concerns, problems, or feelings. Counseling is a learning process that focuses on the personal growth of the parents, who learn to acquire, develop, and utilize the necessary skills and attitudes for resolving their problem or concern. Parents are helped in becoming fully functioning individuals who assist their child and value a well-adjusted family. (pp. 27-28)

The goals of counseling may include helping individuals to work toward an understanding of themselves, to reduce depression, anxiety, guilt, anger, and frustration, and to learn new ways of coping with and adjusting to life situations (Rollin, 1987). Counseling, as practiced by most speech-language pathologists and audiologists, is designed to provide information, to allow clients to explore feelings related to communication disorders and/or treatment, to help and support clients and their families as they change communication or communication-related behaviors, and to help them make the best use of the resources available to them (Stone & Olswang, 1989).

To accomplish these goals, counselors adopt certain attitudes and use certain behaviors that are consistent with their theory or method of counseling. Some theories/methods of counseling include: existential therapy, person-centered therapy, gestalt therapy, behavior therapy, reality therapy, rational-emotive therapy, transactional analysis, and cognitive therapy (Baruth & Huber, 1985). For example, person-centered or Rogerian counselors attempt to maintain an attitude of respect and unconditional acceptance or "positive regard" which allows the client to express and examine his/her feelings and discover any incongruities between his/her perceptions and reality. The counselor facilitates this process by listening to and reflecting or paraphrasing the client's feelings and thoughts while supporting the client emotionally. (See Rodgers [1951] or Rollin [1987] for a more thorough discussion of this topic.)

In contrast, rational-emotive therapists or counselors hold the belief that emotional disturbances result from irrational beliefs and that clients need to be re-educated regarding these beliefs. In rational-emotive therapy (RET), the client expresses feelings and attitudes and the counselor helps him/her to discover irrational attitudes and incongruities by attacking these beliefs and teaching new attitudes (Rollin, 1987).

While there are clear differences between these two counseling techniques and between these and the others not discussed here, there are also similarities found among all good counselors. Good counselors attempt to cultivate an attitude of trust, authenticity, genuineness, and honesty, while trying not to be cold, aloof, or self-righteous (Rollin, 1987). They also attempt to create a therapeutic atmosphere "in which the client feels accepted and recognized as a person who has the potential for change" (Rollin, 1987, p. 17).

To understand counseling as it is practiced by speech-language pathologists and audiologists, it may be helpful to differentiate it from psychotherapy. While these two processes are similar in that they are both designed to help people change, counselors generally work with people who are functioning adequately (in an emotional sense) in their day-to-day activities. Psychotherapists, on the other hand, often work with people who are not coping well with daily life. These people often need to restructure not only their behavior or their thoughts and feelings on a given topic, they need to restructure their personalities (Rollin, 1987) and/or their thought processes.

It may also be helpful to emphasize that the focus of counseling for speech-language pathologists and audiologists is usually on issues related to communication development or disorders or the process of changing communication behaviors (Stone & Olswang, 1989). The focus may be somewhat broader when working with families of high-risk infants or infants and toddlers with impairments because there are so many risk factors which may act as influences on the development of communication (see Chapter 3). Any of these factors may be sources of stress, information need, or difficulty for the family, and may therefore be topics for emphasis in counseling.

In addition to differentiating counseling from psychotherapy and specifying the usual focus for counseling by speech-language-hearing professionals, it may be helpful to discuss the relationship of counseling to family therapy. Like speech-language pathology, counseling and psychotherapy have traditionally focused on the individual. Family therapy, a special form of psychological intervention, developed when some service providers became frustrated with the techniques of individual psychotherapy and began to look at the context within which the psychopathology had developed. Early theorists, such as Satir, Ackerman, Jackson, Haley, Bowen, and Minuchin, were especially interested in the etiology of schizophrenia and the possible role of the family in its development (Foley, 1987).

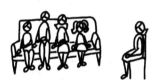

CONJOINT FAMILY THERAPY

This family focus gave rise to a brand of intervention that focuses on the family system rather than the person in it. Family therapy puts the ". . . family in the foreground and the individual member in the background" (Foley, 1987, p. 3). In addition to this readjusted focus, family therapists are concerned with interconnections between family members, the overall pattern of connections within a family, and how these family relationships influence the behavior of each person.

Several models of family therapy have evolved and are discussed by Foley (1987). In conjoint family therapy, the therapist meets with all family members together and focuses on patterns of family interaction. Multiple impact therapy is practiced with several members of a treatment team working with individual family members and various combinations of members intensively for a brief period of time, usually two or three days. In network therapy, the nuclear fam-

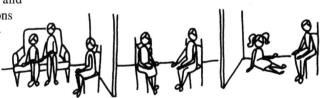

MULTIPLE IMPACT THERAPY

ily, as well as neighbors and friends, meet with a therapist with the goal of forming a "viable social network" for the family (Foley, 1987, p. 4). Finally, in multiple family therapy, several families are seen at once to facilitate observation, imitation, and identification with other families and the development of a relationship between the therapist and the family.

While the general skills or techniques required to practice family therapy are similar to those used in counseling, both the focus on the family and emphasis on family interaction patterns differentiate it from individual treatment. In addition, its emphasis on the family as a system, which was discussed in the early chapters of this book, distinguishes it from other approaches.

NETWORK THERAPY

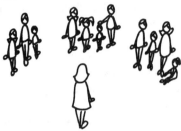

MULTIPLE FAMILY THERAPY

Use of Counseling and Family Therapy Techniques in Family-Centered Early Intervention

The use of counseling skills has long been advocated in speech-language pathology and audiology (Stone & Olswang, 1989). ASHA's (1990) Scope of Practice states that "Speech-language pathologists and audiologists counsel individuals with disorders of communication, their families, caregivers and other service providers relative to the disability present and its management" (p. 1). While it is not the intent of this statement to claim that speech-language pathologists and audiologists should engage in general psychotherapy or in counseling beyond that related to communication and its disorders, it does suggest the importance of counseling to these professions. The work that we do with very young children and their families gives us one of our best opportunities to employ counseling skills.

Several sections of this book have emphasized the broad range of factors that can influence communication development both positively and negatively. The emotional aspects of family members' reactions to and interactions with an infant who has an impairment have also been discussed. These issues, coupled with the sometimes overwhelming amount of information concerning the infant's health and/or developmental status, often precipitate a situation which calls for the creation of a counseling relationship between family members and one or more of the professionals involved with them. Family members often need support and help to cope constructively with all that is "thrown" at them. In addition, when a young child's health and development are at stake, emotions are involved. This may be especially true when communication is at risk. As Luterman (1984) has stated, "Feelings are a large part of the communication process; when communication is defective, affect tends to be high" (pp. 2-3). These feelings are unlikely to resolve or be channeled in a helpful direction without some attention being paid to them.

Speech-language pathologists have to be careful not to assume that their only role relative to families and counseling is to keep an eye out for psychopathology or family dysfunction so that a referral can be made to some other professional. The families who need our help will not necessarily be characterized by psychopathology or dysfunction. They are most likely to be families under stress who need our support to function optimally as a growth medium for their children's communication. We must be prepared both educationally and psychologically to enter into counseling relationships with families of infants and toddlers and to provide this support.

Some Problems with the Use of Counseling

Despite widespread emphasis on the importance of counseling, there are a number of issues related to the use of counseling skills by speech-language pathologists that may have prevented our optimal use of these skills in the past. The first of these issues relates to our profession's conception of what counseling really is and whether and under what circumstances we should be doing it at all. Luterman (1984) points out that the word *counseling* has been used to mean "information-providing and advice giving" (p. 1) as well as, in the definition we are using here, providing a safe, accepting relationship in which the client can examine and perhaps change thoughts, feelings, and behaviors. Practitioners in our profession have generally been comfortable with the information and advice side of counseling while maintaining a more tentative posture in regard to the emotion-related side. While recognizing the difficulty of separating the emotion from communication disorders, most authors have suggested a middle road in counseling for speech-language pathologists. On this middle road, we are to steer clear of clinical behavior that could be labeled "psychotherapy" as well as any subject that is not related to the communication disorder.

Stone and Olswang (1989) have identified professionals' discomfort with counseling as a problem of "poorly defined boundaries" relating to the "range, depth, or style of counseling appropriate for a specialist in communication disorders" (p. 27). These authors have suggested goals, content, and a counseling style that they consider to be within the boundaries of communication specialists.

Another major problem related to use of counseling techniques by speech-language pathologists concerns their training or education to act as counselors. Graduates of training programs in communication science and disorders seldom feel well prepared to do counseling (Luterman, 1984, 1991; Rollin, 1987). With experience, opportunity, and the inclination to do so, we often become skilled counselors, but we seldom begin our careers with as much preparation for counseling as for other forms of clinical management.

Bailey and Simeonsson (1988) express a similar concern with professionals' preparation for working with families in general and specifically with the use of family therapy techniques. They note that even when training programs do include coursework in working with families, there is seldom clinical experience to solidify the skills studied. Because involvement with the families of infants and toddlers is inevitable, it seems incumbent upon us to inform ourselves about this area as best we can. Our practice of family-centered treatment will seldom approximate family therapy as it is carried out by family therapists. We will most often do a form of family intervention which is characterized by greater awareness of the family as a system and increased contact with family members that relates to our own area of competence.

Luterman (1984) has discussed the difficulty our profession has had in reconciling the attitudes of humanistic counseling with the strong behavioral orientation that became popular in the field of communication disorders in the 1960s and 1970s. These two theoretical positions take very different stances relative to the development of human behaviors and attitudes and therapist-client equality in the treatment situation. It is from these differences that Luterman sees difficulties arising. Behaviorists, who see all behaviors as being determined by the consequences of a response to a stimulus, find it hard to accept that constructs such as "self-actualizing drive" (Luterman, 1984, p. 5) can play an important role in treatment.

Perhaps an even more important issue is that of equality, responsibility, and control in the therapeutic relationship. For the behaviorist, the relationship between client and clinician is not an equal one. The clinician takes responsibility for controlling the client's behavior, deciding the course and nature of treatment, etc. The humanist or person-centered therapist attempts to promote an equal relationship with the client, and the client assumes responsibility for the course of therapy within the context of the accepting environment provided by the clinician (Luterman, 1984).

Unless one can reconcile the differences between these schools of thought, it is difficult to practice behaviorally based communication treatment and humanistically based counseling together without feeling a split of allegiances. And because accountability in treatment, which is currently considered so important, is often based on behaviorally based treatment regimens, it is difficult to jetison behavioral techniques without feeling irresponsible or unethical. Further, when we practice person-centered counseling it is difficult to be account-able in terms of stimuli presented percentages of correct responses, etc. Conse-quently, it is and probably will remain difficult to be totally comfortable with counseling in a behaviorally dominated field no matter how well we define our boundaries or master counseling skills.

The Process of Counseling in Family-Centered Early Intervention

Andrews (1986) suggested that clinicians who wish to use family therapy techniques in family-centered intervention need to assess their abilities and attitudes in four areas: "confidence in clinical skills, acceptance of differing points of view, ability to listen, and understanding of the grief process" (p. 347). The family therapy techniques that Andrews (1986) and Andrews and Andrews (1990) recommend for use in treatment of communication disorders are "joining," basic interviewing skills, tracking interactive patterns, clinical testing with family participation, creative strategizing, and task assignment. Andrews and Andrews (1990) describe joining as the process through which "the speech-language pathologist gains acceptance of and admittance into the family system" (p. 90). This process requires demonstrating that the clinician hears and respects what each family member has to say and acknowledges the family's established roles. Family strengths are affirmed. This process, which begins with the first contacts between family and professional, is a process of bonding and forming an alliance (Andrews & Andrews, 1990). Andrews and Andrews suggest adopting the following behaviors to facilitate the joining process: "socializing about everyday issues, mirroring the terminology that matches the family's level of understanding, matching affect (smiling, frown-ing, looking puzzled), and identifying each family member's unique interests and attributes" (p. 91).

Interviewing skills were discussed earlier in this chapter. Those that the Andrews find especially helpful in working with families include attending, clarification (restatement of what the interviewee has said), reflection, and summarizing.

Tracking interactive patterns is a process by which the clinician tries to gather information about communication behavior and the context in which it occurs. Andrews and Andrews (1980) gather this information by asking ques-tions concerning communication behavior and observing interactions that oc-cur as explanations are given. They gather information both from the report given by the family member(s) and from the process of reporting (e.g., the nonverbal communication and flow of information between different family members). They also track interactive patterns when spontaneous communica-tion occurs between family members during the session. Information gathered in this way can help in the process of planning change by providing examples of behaviors that might be increased or decreased.

As the family and clinician come to understand the communication problem and the changes that should occur, creative strategizing can take place. This is the process by which the family and speech-language pathologist decide on ways that family members can facilitate change in the communication behavior. The result of creative strategizing is task assignment.

Once a desired change is defined and a strategy for creating that change is identified, procedures for accomplishing the task are designed. The next step is assigning the task. Andrews and Andrews (1990) suggest that task assignment be preceded by a compliment and delivered in an egalitarian manner (e.g., "Mrs. J., you do a wonderful job of following Jenny's lead in play. You watch to see what she's interested in and you play along with her. How about trying a few statements about what she's doing to give her some words to go with her actions? For example, when you're playing with the ball, you could say, 'Ball. Roll ball. Let's roll the ball.' "

Using these skills, Andrews and Andrews (1986, 1990) propose a "family systems process." This process includes the phases of (1) convening or joining (a process of bringing the family together and enlisting their help in treatment); (2) sharing an understanding of the problem (gathering information on the problem from the family's point of view without disagreeing, offering advice, etc.); (3) agreeing on behaviors to be changed and setting goals (collaborative goal setting with the family's perception of the problem as the focus, sometimes called "creative strategizing"); (4) determining a method of treatment (combining the speech-language pathologist's expertise with knowledge of the family's interaction patterns to select procedures that fit the family. It is important in this phase to preserve ". . . family roles and procedures until their permission is obtained to make adjustments and alterations" (Andrews & Andrews, 1986, p. 363); (5) assessing treatment effectiveness (the family evaluates progress at each session); and finally (6) terminating and linking (a collaborative decision is made to end treatment, and, if necessary, a process of transition to treatment in another setting is facilitated).

EXERCISE #2

Find someone in your locale who does family-centered treatment and arrange to observe in their clinical setting if possible. Make notes on the techniques they use and try some of them in your own clinical work.

CONSULTATION/COLLABORATION

The ability to act as a consultant in a collaborative relationship is of paramount importance to our ability to function as members of early intervention teams. Consultation, as we will use the term here, is an interactive process which is designed to provide technical assistance, skills, knowledge, and training (Gullotta, 1987) to other service providers so that they may facilitate communication growth in infants and toddlers. It is a special service activity in that the consultant does not work directly with the person in need of intervention. Instead, the consultant provides indirect service by sharing information, skills, and support with other professionals, organizations, support personnel, or caregivers who in turn give direct service to the client. This process is especially important in the transdisciplinary model of teaming discussed in Chapter 4.

Frassinelli, Superior, and Meyers (1983) discuss collaborative consultation in the context of the classroom where speech-language pathologists might consult with teachers, but they noted that their model can be applied in other settings such as work with parents. They suggested that three different types of the collaborative model of consultation can be conceptualized depending upon the consultant's degree of direct contact with the client. Degrees of contact range from ongoing direct contact to one-time or periodic contact to no direct contact. Further information on these types of consultation can be found in Table 5-1.

Component Skills

Consultation requires the use of some of the skills that have already been discussed in this chapter, such as interviewing and counseling, as well as an amalgam of problem solving, organizing, and teaching skills (Ehly, Conoley, & Rosenthal, 1985). Perhaps most importantly it requires a firm grasp of the information and skills that can be used to improve an infant's or toddler's ability to acquire and develop adequate communication skills coupled with the expertise to help others to understand, accept, and use what you know. Part of this process is the ability to facilitate another's involvement or motivation (Ehly et al., 1985). Ehly and co-workers discuss seven relationship skills that they consider to be important to the consultation process. Many of these skills parallel those required of a good counselor. These seven skills are: rapport building, empathy, tolerance for individual differences, genuineness, careful listening, flexible problem solving, and feedback skills.

Table 5-1 Types of Collaborative Consultation

Type 1 Ongoing Direct Contact	Combined use of direct treatment and consultation where the consultant has ongoing, direct contact with the infant or toddler and family. The consultant and parent or other professional cooperatively devise activities to facilitate treatment goals. The parent or other professional implements the activities on a day-to-day basis and tracks progress.
Type 2 One-Time or Periodic Contact	Consultation regarding an infant or toddler and family following assessment. Consultation is based on one-time or periodic assessment and re-assessment. The consultant and parent or other professional devise a program which is implemented by the parent or other professional with periodic re-assessment by the consultant.
Type 3 No Direct Contact	Consultation regarding an infant or toddler and family or group of families with infants/toddlers where the consultant has no direct contact with the child(ren). Data collection and observation are done by another professional and the consultant helps to plan a program.

Source: From "A Consultation Model for Speech and Language Intervention" by L. Frassinelli, K. Superior, and J. Meyers, 1983, *ASHA, 25,* p. 27. Copyright 1983 by American Speech-Language-Hearing Association. Adapted by permission.

Use of Consultation Skills in Family-Centered Early Intervention

There are many good reasons to use consultation skills in early intervention, especially as it is to be practiced under P.L. 99-457. Some of the reasons relate to the requirements of the law and available person power to fill these requirements. For example, this law requires that services be delivered by multi-disciplinary teams. Consultation skills can form the basis for the development of efficient collaborative relationships between all team members including family members. In addition, trained personnel from various disciplines who are prepared to work with infants and toddlers are proving to be difficult to find in some states or service delivery districts. Because of this shortage of qualified personnel, the professionals who are well trained in this area may be in demand as consultants.

Other reasons for the use of consultation skills in early intervention relate to the provision of the best services, regardless of requirements or personnel availability. We can act as consultants to the family. Through our role as consultants we can help family members to develop skills to facilitate communication development in their children. By fostering this ability we will help to maintain the natural function of the family in regard to communication development. This, in turn, will provide an opportunity for enhanced self-esteem and perception of competence, especially by parents, and the empowerment that goes with these feelings. The child will also benefit greatly from receiving more continuous help with communication development than any nonresident professional could provide.

The primary problem with speech-language pathologists acting as consultants is our lack of training to do so. While we do get some training in the component skills of consultation, few training programs provide adequate practical experience in consultation either to other professionals or to families. In light of the opportunities that P.L. 99-457 is likely to open, it would seem important for all graduate students to have the chance to gain supervised practice in consultation in various settings and to various populations.

The Process of Consultation

The process of consultation moves through at least four stages. In stage one, or the entry stage, the consultant and the consultee get to know each other and the problem is identified for which the consultant's expertise is needed. This stage often includes negotiation of a contract, establishment of mutual trust, and discussion of mutually acceptable goals for the outcome of the consultation (Cornett & Chabon, 1988; Frassinelli et al., 1983).

Stage two is the time for thorough assessment of the problem. Interviews, observations, and assessments are done with special emphasis on the consultee's perception of the problem. An important component in this assessment should be inquiry into what the consultee has already attempted to do to solve the problem. It is important initially for the consultant not to propose unilaterally derived solutions to the problems (Frassinelli et al., 1983).

In stage three, planning the intervention takes place with both the consultant and consultee contributing ideas, solutions, and establishing priorities. Long-term goals are reviewed and short-term objectives are established. It is important that these goals and objectives be mutually generated and accepted.

Stage four is the time for implementation of the plan. Whatever objectives have been generated in stage three are put into practice.

In the final stage, the success of the intervention process and the consultation itself are evaluated. Progress toward goals is assessed, feedback from the consultee is solicited, and the consultation is terminated (Cornett & Chabon, 1988).

This progression is much like the process of family-based treatment described by Andrews and Andrews (1990). Indeed, the processes both employ the professional's expertise to help in solving a problem while keeping the family or other staff members involved in the solution. The result of consultation as well as family-centered treatment should be a feeling of accomplishment for the consultee(s). As Coufal (1991) states, "People [consultees] should go away feeling as though they solved the problem."

EXERCISE #3

If you are a student enrolled in a practicum or if you are in practice with other professionals, volunteer to consult with one of your colleagues. Make it clear that you are hoping to gain some experience in consultation, rather than requesting a paid position. Role play consultation in the classroom as you did interviewing. Follow the suggestions in this chapter and in the readings referenced. Give each other feedback on your effectiveness as a consultant or consultee.

CONCLUSION

With the mastery of these special skills, professionals will be well prepared for their roles in family-centered intervention. The next section of the book addresses family and child assessment, the first step in the intervention process.

Part III

Preventive Intervention in the Family Context: Assessment and Intervention

The final section of the book presents ideas for evaluating the family in general and as a context for communication development, for evaluating the child as a communicator, and strategies for effective intervention with young children and their families.

6

Assessment of the Family As a Context for Communication Development

Assessment is certainly not a new area of expertise for the communication specialist. Our focus of assessment in the past, however, has almost always been on the communication skills and abilities of the person with the communication problem. As our knowledge of early communication development has grown, we have realized that a complete assessment of a young child's abilities and problems must include an assessment of the environment in which he or she is learning to communicate. We need skills and information that will allow us to look at the family as a context for communication development.

This change in focus is also evident in the requirements of P.L. 99-457 which requires that the strengths and needs of families of handicapped and at-risk children be assessed. Although family assessment is considered a requirement of the law, the final regulations for P.L. 99-457 explain that family assessment is voluntary on the part of the family (*Federal Register,* 1989). The intent of this requirement is for professionals to help the family to focus on what they need in order to assist appropriately in their child's development. "The premise behind this approach is that with the right kind of resources, every family can support the development of a special needs child; the service system is to support, not supplant, the family" (Administration on Developmental Disabilities (ADD), 1988, p. 31).

This change of assessment focus from the child alone to the child as part of a family requires additional skills on the part of early intervention clinicians. This chapter will first consider some of the issues of assessment of family strengths and needs in general, such as why it is necessary, who should participate in the assessment process, what should be assessed, and how the assessment can be achieved. It is not intended that the coverage of this topic be exhaustive. In general, speech-language pathologists will not be solely responsible for aiding in the assessment of the family concerns, priorities, and resources. The information is presented in sufficient detail for the reader to participate knowledgeably in general family assessment. For a more complete treatment of the topic, see Bailey and Simeonsson (1988) or McGonigel, Kaufmann, and Johnson (1991).

The terms *family assessment* and *identification of family strengths and needs* are both used in P.L. 99-457. Because both families and professionals have become concerned that family assessment by professionals may be an intrusive activity, it has been emphasized that it is the professional's role to assist the family in self-assessment. Some professionals and families prefer the term *identification of the concerns, priorities, and resources* to *family assessment* (Kaufman & McGonigel, 1991). The terms will be used interchangeably here.

The second section will address the specific issues involved in assessment of the family as a communicative environment for the language-learning child. This topic is treated in greater detail because this specific aspect of identification of family strengths and needs is particularly the domain of the speech-language pathologist.

ASSESSMENT OF STRENGTHS AND NEEDS OF THE FAMILY SYSTEM

The earlier chapters of this book described the family's function as a system. Family assessment can consider the various components of that system or its general function as a whole. Bailey (1991) defines family assessment as "the ongoing and interactive process by which professionals gather information in order to determine family priorities for goals and services . . . family assessment is a continuous process involving both family members and professionals" (p. 27). The goal of this assessment is for "professionals to understand what families want for themselves and their children and what they need from professionals in order to achieve those aspirations" (p. 27).

Need for Family Assessment

There are many reasons to change our assessment focus to include the family. Our reasons for carrying out such an evaluation will influence how we conduct the evaluation. If our reason for evaluation is to "find out what's wrong with a family," our efforts may be perceived as intrusive or threatening by family members. If our focus is only on identifying family needs and deficits we may make the family feel like a "bag of problems." If our reason for evaluation is, instead, to help the family find out what family strengths and resources can be martialed, enhanced, and supported to help the child, and what a family needs to be most able to help the child, family members may be able to function as true members of the evaluation team, participating fully in the assessment procedures.

Bailey (1991) has offered definitions of "strengths" and "needs" as the terms relate to family assessment. "*Family need* may be viewed as a family's ex-

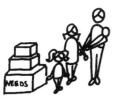 pressed desire for services to be obtained or outcomes to be achieved. A *family strength* is the family's perception of resources that are at its disposal that could be used to meet family needs" (p. 27). He further emphasizes that in terms of P.L. 99-457, a need exists only if a family member perceives it and expresses a desire for services in that area. Professionals may, of course, assist families in identifying needs, but they should not make ". . . overt or covert attempts to force families to recognize needs they do not perceive to exist" (p. 30). Likewise, if family members perceive needs that professionals do not believe to be very important, professionals should respect and attend to those perceived needs. As Bailey states, "If professionals initially focus on family-expressed priorities, families are likely to develop a sense of ownership and feelings of trust" (p. 31). Dunst, Trivette, and Deal (1988) express a similar belief when they counsel professionals to "start *where the family is,* beginning with the things that are important to the family unit. . . . " This idea will be explored further in Chapter 8.

Bailey and Simeonsson (1988) list five reasons to assess families:

1. to meet legal mandates, specifically requirements of P.L. 99-457
2. to understand a child as part of a family system in which intervention with the child may affect the rest of the family in either helpful or stressful ways
3. to identify families' needs for services such as information about the disability, help in locating day care, or help in interacting with the child
4. to identify families' strengths that promote family adaptation such as support from family members, friends, or organizations
5. to expand the base for evaluating services by establishing a baseline measure against which to assess change.

Who Should Be Included in the Family?

If all families were traditional, nuclear families, there would be no need for this question. But functioning family units frequently include members other than mom, dad, and the kids. As noted in Chapter 1, relatives, friends, mother's boyfriend, or day care personnel may spend large amounts of time with the child and consequently may influence the child's development. It may be important to include all of these influential people in the family assessment process. Those to be included will often depend on the ethnic or cultural circumstances of the family. In some cultures, for example, grandparents are important sources of advice to young parents and consequently need to be included in the assessment process (ADD, 1988; Hanson et al., 1990).

What Should Be Assessed?

Many facets of the family system may be important to the development of a child and his or her communication skills. Trivette, Deal, and Dunst (1986) suggested that the family functions (i.e., financial, physical, vocational, recreational, educational, emotional, and cultural/social) provide a useful framework for assessing family needs which are related to these functions.

Bailey and Simeonsson (1988) cite five domains for family assessment:

1. child needs and characteristics likely to affect family functioning
2. parent-child interactions
3. family needs
4. critical events
5. family strengths (p. 10)

Child needs and characteristics that should be assessed might include the child's behavior and temperament, responsiveness, repetitive behaviors, or unusual caregiving demands. Aspects of parent-child interaction that might be considered in this part of the evaluation include how parents teach the child or read and respond to his or her behaviors, as well as the positive or negative tone of the interactions and the evidence of an emotional bond between the child and parents. (Interaction as it relates specifically to communication development will be discussed later in this chapter.) Family needs might relate to financial responsibilities, isolation, information, stress, etc. Critical events to be aware of might include the initial diagnosis, medical crises, or failure to attain developmental milestones at expected times. The assessment of family strengths might include consideration of personal or family resources as well as sources of support outside the family, such as from church or community organizations. In addition to these five domains, the home environment in general may need to be considered (Bailey & Simeonsson, 1988).

It is important to note that family strengths are evaluated as part of the family assessment. One cautionary statement has been made concerning the consideration of strengths. There may be some danger, especially in programs where costs are high and funds are scarce, of using the documentation of family strengths as justification for denial of services (ADD, 1988). For example, a family that is considered to have good resources for handling stress may not be provided with the option to receive counseling, even though some members of the family might be better able to promote the at-risk child's development if those services were provided. The intent of evaluation of strengths is, of course, to be aware of the family's abilities that may be promoted and used to work on other less strong areas.

Ways To Identify Family Concerns, Priorities, and Resources

Important Considerations

Current thinking emphasizes the importance of realizing that the family is the best evaluator of its own needs (ADD, 1988; Bailey, 1991; Kaufmann & McGonigel, 1991). This does not mean that families always come to the intervention situation with well-defined ideas of what they need and want for services or even what services may be available. Frequently, families can benefit from the help of a number of professionals in identifying and expressing their needs and strengths. However, the evaluation must fit the needs of the family rather than the needs of the program. For example, even though the program may not have an occupational therapist (OT) on staff, if the child needs to be evaluated by an OT, an evaluation by that professional should be made available (ADD, 1988). The staffing of the program should not determine the needs of the family.

Bailey and Simeonsson (1988) have listed six characteristics of effective family assessment. The assessment must:

1. cover important family domains
2. incorporate multiple sources and measures
3. recognize the importance of family values and traditions
4. determine family priorities for goals and services
5. vary according to program type and demands
6. evaluate family outcomes on a regular basis (p. 9)

The domains mentioned in the first assessment characteristic are discussed in the section above. Multiple sources of information will be provided in part by the different professionals involved, and in part by the use of different measures.

The recognition of family values, especially culturally based values, and traditions can often mean the difference between success and failure in the family-professional relationship. The more a family perceives its values to be common to, or at least accepted by, the professionals with whom they deal, the more comfortable they may be relating to those people. If they feel disapproval, or if they disapprove of the professional's values, difficulties may arise. If planned treatments or goals do not fit with their values, the program may fail.

As Bailey and Simeonsson (1988) state, "If early interventionists fail to recognize strong family values and attempt to implement services or goals that conflict with those values, the inevitable result is mistrust and failure to follow through" (p. 15).

For example, it is sometimes important for professionals to accept and support the use of folk or herbal remedies in addition to more modern methods of treatment if families are convinced of their efficacy. As another example, it may be important to recognize family tradition as a factor in determining the time table for some approaches to feeding infants. In families in which babies "always take solid foods by four months," it may be futile to insist that attempts to include solids be delayed until some later age.

Kaufmann and McGonigel (1991) present seven principles summarizing important concerns for identifying family concerns, priorities, and resources (see Exhibit 6-1).

To be effective, family assessment must determine family priorities for goals and services. The family's perceived needs must become first priority goals for treatment (ADD, 1988; Bailey & Simeonsson, 1988; Kaufmann & McGonigel, 1991). The type of program (i.e., center- or home-based) that will be available to the child and family is another consideration in determining the content of the family assessment. Parents who are to provide direct intervention for the child in the home may need quite different skills from those needed by parents

---

Exhibit 6-1 Principles for Identifying Family Concerns, Priorities, and Resources

- The inclusion of family information in the IFSP is voluntary on the part of the families.
- The identification of family concerns, priorities, and resources is based on an individual family's determination of which aspects of family life are relevant to the child's development.
- A family need or concern exists only if the family perceives that the need or concern exists.
- Families have a broad array of formal and informal options to choose from in determining how they will identify their concerns, priorities, and resources.
- Families have multiple and continuing opportunities to identify their concerns, priorities, and resources.
- Family confidences are respected, and family-shared information is not discussed casually among staff.
- The process of identifying family concerns, priorities, and resources leads to the development of IFSP outcomes, strategies, and activities that help families achieve the things they want from early intervention for their children and themselves.

Source: From *Guidelines and Recommended Practices for the Individualized Family Service Plan,* 2nd ed. (p. 50) by M. McGonigel, R. Kaufmann, and B. Johnson (eds.). Bethesda, MD: Association for the Care of Children's Health.

who will be primarily responsible for generalization of skills learned in a center-based program. The assessment must be tailored to uncover these fine differences in abilities (Bailey & Simeonsson, 1988).

The family assessment must be updated at regular intervals, at least every six months, to reflect changes in family strengths and needs. Such ongoing evaluations can both document program successes or failures related to family goals and discover additional characteristics that may be resources or areas of need for intervention (Bailey & Simeonsson, 1988).

Another issue concerning the family assessment may be the number of sessions devoted to the evaluation process. Cost-conscious programs may attempt to accomplish this process in as few sessions as possible. Several authors (e.g., Fraiberg, 1980; Trout, 1987; Westby, 1988) suggest that rushing the family assessment may be counterproductive. Assessment occurs during the earliest contacts between the family and the professionals and as such is the time when these important team members work out their relationships and roles. Time is required for trust to develop and for a working relationship to evolve. Both Fraiberg (1980) and Trout (1987) suggest that at least five sessions be planned for assessment and that the evaluators be the same people who will work with the family over time.

Some Available Measures

Bailey (1991) notes that every interaction between family members and professionals is actually part of the assessment process. Every phone call, visit, appointment, question asked or answered, or other interaction provides an opportunity for information gathering. In Bailey's opinion, "the value of these opportunities for information gathering is substantial, and when possible, they should form the core of any family assessment component" (p. 27). He further notes that family members tend to prefer this kind of informal approach to family assessment.

Bailey and Simeonsson (1988) suggest the use of three kinds of measures when more formal assessment is required: (1) tests, survey instruments, and rating forms; (2) naturalistic observation; and (3) interviews.

Tests, survey instruments, and rating forms. Tests, survey instruments, and rating forms can be used to help family members identify their concerns and resources. It should be emphasized that these measures are not designed to "test" families or to provide information that will be used to compare one family with another. Measures that are recommended for use in family assessment do not include psychological instruments to measure such variables as stress, personality characteristics, etc., unless family members specifically request help in assessing such factors. The measures that are suggested can be used for self-assessment by family members, either privately or with one or more professionals, or as a guide for an interview conducted by a professional, depending upon the family's preference. These measures may help families to identify concerns or resources which they might otherwise overlook (Bailey, 1991; Kaufmann & McGonigel, 1991). See Exhibit 6-2 for a list of written measures which may be useful for family assessment.

The way in which the measure is used with the family may be as important as the measure chosen. Dunst et al. (1988) suggest the following four steps be taken when a survey-type measure is used in family assessment. (1) Explain why you want the family to complete the scale (e.g., "Your answers to these questions may help us all to identify areas where we might be able to help you with some problem or need"). (2) Clarify how the results will be used (e.g., "We'll talk with you about your answers to get a better idea of the things you need. There are no right or wrong answers, and your responses won't be compared with anyone else's"). (3) Use the responses to clarify and define family needs (e.g., "You have indicated that you need help finding day care for your child. Tell me more about the days and times when you need child care"). (4) Restate the needs as you understand them (e.g., "If I understand correctly, the things you'd most like help with are finding day care, learning how to help Julio learn to talk, and finding time to spend with your other children).

Naturalistic observation. Naturalistic observation may also be used to assess various aspects of parent-child interaction. By using videotape, family members can participate with professionals in observing their own interactions to look for behaviors that are especially helpful to their child or that make it difficult for their child to accomplish desired goals. This kind of assessment can be used to define specific needs related to the caregiving environment. The second section of this chapter suggests one way that this kind of naturalistic observation could be used to assess the communicative environment provided by a family for a child who is at risk for speech and/or language deficits. Other measures are available for evaluating parent-child interactions by means of structured observation. Nine of these measures are listed and briefly described in Exhibit 6-3.

Exhibit 6-2 Written Measures for Family Assessment

- Family Needs Survey, Revised Edition (Bailey & Simeonsson, 1990)
- Parent Needs Survey (Darling, 1988)
- Family Needs Scale (Dunst, Cooper, Weeldreyer, Synder, & Chase, 1988)
- Family Support Scale (Dunst, Jenkins, & Trivette, 1988)
- Exercise: Social Support (Summers, Turnbull, & Brotherson, 1985)
- Prioritizing Family Needs Scale (Finn & Vadasy, 1988)

Exhibit 6-3 Measures of Parent-Child Interaction

- The Dyadic Mini Code (Censullo, M., Bowler, R., Lester, B., & Brazelton, T.B., 1987). This instrument is designed to measure adult-infant interaction synchrony from video-taped interaction.
- The Greenspan-Lieberman Observation System (GLOS) (Greenspan, S. & Lieberman, A., 1980).
  The GLOS provides a micro-analytic technique for assessing parent and child verbal and nonverbal behaviors.
- Observation of Communicative Interaction (OCI) (Klein, M. & Briggs, M., 1986).
  The OCI provides a framework for considering ten kinds of desirable maternal behaviors that may be used in mother-infant interaction in a check sheet format.
- Ecoscales Manual (MacDonald, J., Gillette, Y., & Hutchinson, T., 1989).
  The Ecoscales are designed to be used to analyze adult and child interactive and communicative skills and to establish treatment goals.
- Diagnostic Interaction Survey (Owens, R., 1982).
  The DIS is designed to identify parent-child interaction behaviors including reinforcement/punishment, nonverbal cues, conversation, verbal cues, and child register.
- The Maternal (Parent) Behavior Rating Scale (Mahoney, G., Powell, A., & Finger, I., 1986).
  This scale is designed to look at eight aspects of parent behavior in order to assess the quality of parent-child interaction.
- Interaction Analysis Chart (McDade, H. & Simpson, M., 1984).
  This chart provides ten categories for scoring parent communicative behaviors and four categories for scoring child behaviors.
- Objective Observation Tool for Parent-Child Interaction (Russo, J. & Owens, R., 1982).
  This tool is a ten-item taxonomy designed to assess parent and child interaction behaviors.
- Parent Behavior Progression (Bromwich, R., Khokha, E., Fust, L., Baxter, E., Burge, D., & Kass, E., 1981).
  Assesses infant-related maternal behaviors, such as apparent pleasure in proximity to infant, and ability to read infant cues.

Rosenberg, Robinson, and Beckman (1986) suggested that measures such as these should:

(1) permit reliable assessment of dyads containing young children whose patterns of behavior may be ambiguous due to a handicap that limits the child's ability to interact; (2) offer a system that is efficient and that can be easily incorporated into an intervention program; and (3) identify strategies that foster effective interaction between parents and their young handicapped children. (pp. 35-36)

They also note that a clinician who is selecting an interaction measure for use should consider the measure's content (is it consistent with the parenting skills or style that the clinician wishes to foster?), its reliability (inter-rater and internal consistency) and sensitivity to changes in behavior, and its practicality of use.

Interviews. Public Law 99-457 specifies that family assessment must be based on "information provided by the family through a personal interview" (*Federal Register* 54, p. 26320). Consequently, even when some other measure is used to aid the family in identifying their concerns, priorities, and resources, a formal or informal interview must be conducted.

Information on interviewing from Patton (1980) is summarized in the chapter on special skills for working with families. Westby (1988) uses Patton's interview categories to classify family assessment interview techniques into four categories: (1) closed, quantitative interviews; (2) standardized, open-ended interviews; (3) interview guides; and (4) informal conversational or ethnographic interviews. Westby suggests that interview guides, which typically consist of a checklist of items that are designed to explore a particular theme using an interview format, and informal conversational or ethnographic interviews, which have no predetermined questions or answer choices, are especially useful in interviewing families.

Turnbull and Turnbull (1986) developed a *Family Assessment Interview Guide* containing questions concerning family resources, family interactions, family functions, and family life cycle. This interview guide is quite detailed and provides many suggestions for interview content which may be especially helpful for the novice interviewer. The following sample questions are from the four sections of this guide:

Family Resources:
- How often do you have contact with extended family members? How do they help you with your child with an exceptionality? (p. 359)
- In general, how does your family approach problems? What helps you most when you are facing difficulty? (p. 360)

Family Interactions:
- What are your feelings and thoughts about your child with an exceptionality? Do you have any unanswered questions or unresolved needs in relation to this child? (p. 360)
- Do people in your family generally support an individual family member in pursuing some goal or interest? How do they show their support? (p. 361)

Family Functions:
- How are chores divided in your family? (Who does the housework, child care, etc.?) Which chores are children expected to perform? Are you satisfied with the way chores are divided? (p. 361)
- What does your family do for fun? (p. 361)

Family Life Cycle:
- What do you think your life and other members of your family's lives will be like 5 years from now? Ten years from now? (p. 362)
- What worries you most about the future? (p. 362)

One of the family assessment surveys discussed above might also be used as an interview guide. If family members have already responded to the survey, items that they indicated as areas of concern or need might be further explored in an interview where they could clarify and specify important issues.

The informal conversational interview may prove to be the most helpful form of interview when used by a skilled interviewer. Dunst et al. (1988) reiterate that the purpose of the interview is to help the family to identify its needs, resources, and priorities, not to convince them of professional opinions on these matters. These authors list seven operatives for the family needs interview

1. Be positive and proactive in arranging the first contact with the family.
2. Take time to establish rapport with the family before beginning the interview.
3. Begin by clearly stating the purpose of the interview.
4. Encourage the family to share aspirations as well as concerns.
5. Help the family clarify concerns, and define the precise nature of their needs.
6. Listen empathetically and be responsive throughout the interview.
7. Establish consensus regarding the priority needs, projects, etc. (p. 66)

The topic of interviewing is covered more completely in Chapter 5.

Possible Problems with Family Assessment

Perhaps the greatest barrier to valid family assessment is the family itself. Without very skillful work on the part of the professional, family members often perceive attempts at uncovering their strengths and needs as intrusive and threatening. Parents especially may fear evaluation of their parenting techniques, home environment, relationships, and support systems. Economic problems may leave little energy to deal with the finer points of child development that may seem to them to be low priority issues (Bailey & Simeonsson, 1988). If parents are still mourning the "loss of the perfect child" or are depressed for other reasons, they may be unable to cooperate adequately with the professionals whose job it is to help them to identify concerns, priorities, and resources (Bailey & Simeonsson, 1988).

Westby (1988) suggests that another potential problem may be averted if consideration is given to the question of who does the evaluation in light of the culture of the family to be assessed. In some cultures, for example, younger professionals (in their 20s) are not considered to be wise enough to be given certain kinds of information. Consequently, an evaluator in that age range may not be entrusted with information necessary to the evaluation, and the evaluation results may be invalid. While this seems unfair, it is an important consideration in choice of team members for carrying out the assessment.

The scheduling of the evaluation may pose another potential problem. Although most professionals prefer to work regular business hours, those hours may not be the most convenient times for a family to participate in their evaluation. It may be necessary to schedule evaluation times for evening or weekend hours in order to see all of the important family members (ADD, 1988).

The Administration on Developmental Disabilities (1988) discusses the importance of some of these factors for the assessment of the family required by P.L. 99-457 as follows: "Perhaps more than any other aspect of this legislation, it will take wisdom to navigate between the good of having families be part of the evaluation component, and the dangers of inappropriate intrusions. . . . The key will certainly be in the degree to which parents sense the equal partnership and collaboration with professionals for the child's benefits that the law intends" (p. 32).

Perhaps one of the most important ways to make the family assessment process appropriate and nonintrusive is to try to become aware of the family's preferences. Some families may be capable of taking the lead in identifying their strengths and needs. They may welcome their role as equal partners in the assessment process. Other families may prefer to work with professionals whose expertise they respect and whom they expect to guide them in this aspect of the intervention process.

Bailey (1991) suggests five strategies for reducing the chance that families will find the assessment process intrusive:

1. Make sure that family members understand that the family assessment is optional and that their participation is voluntary.

2. Chose the most practical, nonintrusive, relevant, and least formal measures available. (When possible, ask family members what kind of measure they think would be most helpful.)

3. Make sure that terminology used in assessment tools and interviews is straightforward and positive.

4. Be sensitive to cultural expectations concerning acceptable professional behavior and respectful treatment.

5. Assure and inform family members of the confidentiality of the information they share.

The next section discusses a specific aspect of family assessment, the consideration of the communicative environment that the family provides for its members who are learning language.

ASSESSMENT OF THE COMMUNICATIVE ENVIRONMENT

Children who are engaged in the process of speech and language learning are dependent upon people, experiences, and communication events to fuel this process. All of the factors that provide input to the language-learning process can be considered part of the communicative environment of the child. For some children, this environment is a rich source of stimulation, encouragement, opportunity, and reinforcement for attempts at communication. For others, the speech and language in the environment may be difficult to use as input to the language-learning process for a number of different reasons, or the opportunity and/or rewards for communication attempts may be few. For some children, the characteristics of the environment may not be of prime importance. These children seem to be resilient enough to do reasonably well even under less-than-optimal conditions. For others, especially children who are at risk for language and speech disorders, optimal environmental conditions may be needed to support their development. When children have difficulty in learning speech and/or language, it is sometimes important to assess certain aspects of the family as a context for language learning as a first step to helping the family create a more nearly optimal environment.

Sometimes differences in communicative environments are easy to discern. For example, Mrs. Green addresses her two-year-old boy: "What are you looking at over there? I'm trying to play this game with you. Come on. This is blue. Say blue. Say blue." However, Mrs. Lane's speech to her two-year-old boy is quite different: "Oh you're looking under the table, aren't you. What do you see there? A ball. You see a ball. Let's get that pretty ball."

While there are apparent differences in these two samples, to create a more optimal environment we first must be able to describe the current environment in some objective way. We must also be able to obtain baseline measures of the characteristics of the environment to which we can compare measures taken during treatment.

It should be noted that no argument is being made here for or against the communicative behaviors of the child's partners (usually the parents and other family members) as causes of language-learning or other communication problems. Whatever the cause of the communication problem, the communicative environment may play a role in precipitating, exacerbating, or maintaining the problem, or it may contribute to the process of remediation. It may also be possible to maximize characteristics of this environment so that they help to prevent the development of communication problems.

This section presents various techniques for analyzing the communication behavior of the people with whom the language-learning child interacts. For the purposes of the analysis, this verbal and nonverbal communication behavior is seen as playing two primary roles: (1) it acts as a language model for the child to imitate or at least to process as part of the raw materials for building his or her theory of the way the language works; and (2) it provides consequences for the child's attempts at communication. In addition to having these two major functions, the communication partner's behaviors are characterized by time factors which may affect the child's ability to benefit from the language model or consequences, or the child's ability to attempt to communicate. In addition, the various components of the communication partner's behavior are discussed, and techniques presented for assessing the communication behaviors as they function as a model, as consequences, and for assessing the related time factors.

The Communicative Environment

Every family creates and maintains its own communicative environment for each of its members. This environment consists of all the communication behavior that involves or occurs around the family member. The behaviors include experiences that involve communication (e.g., family birthday parties) where people interact in various ways that involve both verbal and nonverbal communication. Specific communication events may involve one or more family members and/or nonmembers. They may directly involve the child, or simply occur within his or her visual or auditory range.

It should be noted that the family's communicative environment may be experienced differently by different family members. For example, the first-born child may receive a great deal of verbal attention from adults, while later-born children, especially in large families, may interact more with other children.

It is within the communicative environment that children learn to communicate. This environment provides input to the language-learning process in the form of stimuli, language models, and consequences for attempts at communication in the form of reinforcement, feedback, and enhanced need and desire. Research in the area of parent-child interaction with both normal and deficient language learners has shown that several aspects of the communicative environment are especially important to language learning (see Chapter 3). These are the behaviors to be addressed by this evaluation.

The Purpose of Assessment

It should be stressed that the purpose of the evaluation of these aspects of the child's environment is not to find out what's wrong with current patterns of interaction so that the clinician can counsel parents to stop using some offending behavior. The purpose is, instead, to look for positive behaviors or conditions that can be increased. While research has pointed to some behaviors that seem to be helpful for many children, not all children may benefit from the same behaviors. Evaluation must be an individualized process that searches out "what works" for each child in each communication relationship. We are searching for ways to enhance the communicative environment, to make it a more nurturing context for communication growth for both the child and other family members. Our goal is to support the family's ability to provide the communicative environment needed by a particular child. No one should experience the evaluation process as punitive or degrading.

In addition to taking care not to emphasize what's wrong with a communicative environment, we must be careful not to assume that there is one right kind of environment for all children of all cultures, socioeconomic levels, etc. Nurturing communicative environments vary with culture, occupation and education level of the parents, characteristics of the child or other family members, etc. Families with many different communication styles can provide optimal conditions for communication growth. Also, adults in some cultural groups are not likely to converse with young children (e.g., the southeastern black community observed by Heath, 1982), but do still provide a rich linguistic environment for children (Shieffelin & Eisenberg, 1984). If the communicative environment is to be assessed, it must be assessed by someone who is familiar with the communication norms for the family's culture. The information provided in this section of the chapter is most applicable to middle-class American norms of parent-child interaction. It might be argued, however, that if the family's goal is for their child to function in mainstream American society, it may be useful for the family to provide a communicative environment that is similar to the one typical of that society.

To use information on the communicative environment as a basis for treatment planning we must be able to quantify our observations. It is not enough to make global statements about this aspect of family-child interaction. We need specific information and baseline measures. With this quantitative material we can objectively evaluate the family's input and response to the child. The remainder of this chapter presents a framework for observation and quantification of the communicative environment.

Communicative Environment Assessment Techniques

The assessment techniques presented here are organized into three general categories: techniques to assess the language model; techniques for assessment of the consequences of the child's attempts at communication; and assessment of time factors. For each assessment technique, a description, procedure, formula, and ideas on interpretation are given. At the end of the chapter, an example is given to illustrate the use of the techniques.

The measures to be used in the evaluation protocol are designed to look at existing conditions at the time of evaluation. Measures are generally used on samples of communication collected from dyads of family members (e.g., the toddler and mother, the toddler and older brother), but they may also be used on samples of triadic communication (e.g., the toddler and mother and father).

The evaluation techniques in this protocol were selected based on information from the literature on facilitative language input to language-learning children (e.g., Cross, 1984; Snow, 1984) as well as clinical experience. The techniques that have been included focus on behaviors that my colleagues and I have seen repeatedly in parents of speech- or language-impaired children, behaviors that can be changed, and behaviors that when changed, seem to facilitate child speech or language change (Guitar, Kopff, Donahue-Kilburg, & Bond, in press; Kilburg, 1985).

For some of the measures there are normative data that allow comparison of case data to norms. For other measures there are no norms per se, only empirically based estimates of levels that are useful to development. All of the measures become more meaningful as they are re-used to gain a picture of communication change in the family system. While comparison to norms helps the evaluator to identify possible areas of strength and weakness in the communicative environment, it's important not to fall into the pattern of stressing what's wrong with the way Mom talks to Billy, but instead to identify areas of adequacy and strength.

In some cases it may be desirable to use all or most of the separate procedures in the protocol to evaluate one or more dyads in a family. In most cases, however, a quick review of the communication samples will give the evaluator an idea of which measures are important for a particular dyad and only a select few will need to be used. This process of selecting specific measures helps to limit the amount of time required for completion of the assessment.

Obtaining an Interaction Sample

Before any assessment techniques can be used, a sample of language must be collected from any of the persons who interact with the child for whom the clinician wishes to do an assessment. The sample should consist of 50 to 100

adult or older child
utterances collected
while the family
member is interact-
ing with the child.
For all of the meas-
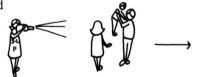
ures discussed here, an utterance is considered to be a unit of speech
terminated by a pause or by an apparent terminal (rising or falling)
intonation contour (Miller, 1981). Child utterances should also be collected so
that comparisons and judgments concerning pragmatic and semantic content
can be made.

Recording and Transcribing the Language/Interaction Sample

Videotaping the sample allows for analysis of nonverbal interaction which is
needed for some measures. The sample can be transcribed in standard orthogra-
phy on a form such as the one in Exhibit 6-4. There is space for notation of
nonverbal as well as verbal behaviors. Once the sample is transcribed, measures can be chosen from the following protocol, and the analysis can be
completed. Appendix 6-A contains a case illustration with examples of the
measures from the protocol.

Assessing the Language Model

When we assess the language model that is available to the child in the
family context we gain insight into the ease with which the child can "tune in"
to the language code used in his or her culture. While it's not practical to
attempt to assess all aspects of the model, it is possible to consider several
components. We can organize the language components into categories of
content, form, and use.

Content

Under the heading of language content, we consider the semantic information in the language model. We want to know what kind of sample of vocabulary is available and how easy it is for the child to link up words and referents.
Two areas of the language model can readily be assessed: vocabulary diversity/
redundancy and reference. For each of these areas, techniques for assessment
are given below.

Vocabulary Diversity/Redundancy. This area of language content can be
assessed by calculating a Type Token Ratio (TTR) (Miller, 1981) for a sample

Exhibit 6-4 Form for Recording Interaction Sample

Child Vocal/Verbal	Child (→) or Adult (←) Nonverbal	Adult Vocal/Verbal

of language collected from one of the child's communication partners. The TTR is an easily computed measure of vocabulary diversity or variability. The ratio of the number of different words (types) to the total number of words (tokens) for a given sample is computed.

Procedure

1. Count all of the words in the sample (tokens); brief rules for counting words (see Miller, 1981, for more):
   - contractions of subject and predicate count as two words (e.g., we're)
   - contractions of verb and negative count as one word (e.g., don't)
   - bound morphemes and noun and verb inflections do not count as separate words

2. Go back through the sample and count each different word (type). While this is not a difficult task, it can be confusing trying to remember which words have already appeared and which have not. Using a form such as that presented in Exhibit 6-5 where each type is placed in a chart alphabetically can make the task easier.

3. Divide the number of types by the number of tokens (Miller, 1981).

Formula

$$\text{Number of types} \div \text{number of tokens} = \text{TTR}$$

Interpretation

A value of 0.50 is generally considered a "normal" TTR, but the larger the sample, the smaller the TTR tends to be (Hess, Sefton, & Landry, 1986). TTR has been found to decrease when adults talk to low-verbal, retarded children

Exhibit 6-5 Type Token Ratio Analysis Form

and to persons having difficulty comprehending language due to distorted transmission (Broen, 1972). Mothers of language-learning children have been shown to use a lower TTR with younger children (Broen, 1972; Chapman, 1979). Chapman (1979) reports a range of TTR scores from 0.31 to 0.53 in studies of mothers' speech to children 8 to 30 months old.

Given this information, but taking into account size of the language sample, a TTR below 0.50 may indicate a helpful adjustment to facilitate comprehension of language content.

Reference: Percentage of "Here-and-Now" Utterances. Children most readily learn words that refer to something in the immediate environment to which they and the caregiver can jointly attend. Therefore, the percent of caregiver utterances that refer to things or events that are present or ongoing here and now may give us an indication of the ease or difficulty the child will have tuning-in to the referent.

Procedure
1. Count the total number of adult utterances.
2. Go back and count each utterance that refers to things or events in the immediate environment.
3. Divide the number of here-and-now utterances by the total number of utterances and multiply by 100 to find the percent.

Formula
Number of here-and-now utterances ÷ number of total utterances × 100 =
percentage of here-and-now utterances

Interpretation
Cross (1977) found this variable to be related to a child's psycholinguistic ability and age with 73 percent of mothers' utterances being here-and-now related. The less linguistically capable and younger the child, the higher the percentage of here-and-now utterances the mother used. Snow (1984) reported 73 to 96 percent here-and-now utterances for mothers of children between 11 and 24 months. A high percentage of here and now utterances (upwards of 65 percent) in the adult model would seem to facilitate language learning.

Form

Another aspect of the language model to which the child is exposed is its form. Components of language form include syntax, morphology, and phonology, the structural aspects of language. Some of the most important aspects of language form as it relates to the child's ability to benefit from the language model are syntactic complexity, syntactic and phonologic integrity and clarity, and the variety of sentence types used.

When we consider language form as input, we want to know whether the model is complex enough to stimulate progress with syntactic development without being too complex for the child to process. We also may be concerned with the clarity of presentation of the model and whether it is clear enough for the child to process and use as a phonological model.

Syntactic Complexity. The syntactic or grammatical complexity of the language model that the child hears from any given communication partner can be assessed by calculating the mean length of utterance (MLU) (Miller, 1981) for a sample of language. This measure gives an easy assessment of the average number of morphemes used by a speaker in a sentence, and consequently reflects the length and complexity of the sentences to which the child is exposed. The measure can be used to compare the partner's complexity to that of the child. Because a comparison will be made, the partner's MLU must be calculated by the same rules used for the child.

Procedure

The following rules for counting morphemes in the utterances of young children were developed by Brown (1973) and adapted by Owens (1988). The same rules should be used for the adult model.

Rule	Example	Morpheme
Count as one morpheme:		
[Each] reoccurrence of a word for emphasis	No, no, no	3
Compound words (two or more free morph.)	Railroad	1
Proper names	Roger Brown	1
Ritualized reduplications	Bye-bye	1
Irregular past tense verbs	Went	1
Diminutives	Doggie	1
Auxiliary verbs and catenatives	Is, hafta	1
Count as two morphemes (inflected verbs and nouns):		
Possessive nouns	Tom's	2
Plural nouns	cats	2
Third person singular present-tense verbs	walks	2
Regular past-tense verbs	walked	2
Present progressive verbs	walking	2
Do not count:		
Disfluencies (count only most complete form of word)	un-undo	1
Fillers	Um, oh, ah	0

After counting the morphemes in each utterance, add the total number of morphemes in the whole sample (at least 50 utterances). Then divide that total by the number of utterances for the MLU.

Formula

Total number of morphemes ÷ total number of utterances = MLU

Interpretation

A number of studies have found that mothers of language-learning children typically adjust their sentence length to an MLU of about 2.4 morphemes longer than the child's (Chapman, 1979). Some studies have also found that mothers of language-disordered children fail to make this adjustment and continue to use much longer utterances which may be difficult for the child to comprehend or imitate (Cross, 1984). Therefore, an adult MLU of more than 3.0 morphemes longer that the child's may be an indication that the language model is too syntactically complex.

Syntactic and Phonologic Integrity and Clarity. Several measures, percent utterances containing disfluent speech, percent utterances containing unintelligible speech, and percent utterances which are grammatically correct, relate to the clarity of the model presented to the child. The fewer disfluencies and episodes of unintelligible speech and the higher the percentage of completely grammatical utterances, the more closely the language model resembles the "ideal."

Procedure and Formulas

To compute the percentage for each of these variables, follow the same procedure used to figure the percentage of here-and-now utterances above.

Number of utterances with disfluencies ÷ number of total utterances × 100 =
percentage utterances with disfluency

(Use the same kind of formula for the other measures.)

Interpretation

Please note that the author seldom uses these measures with the communication partners because they are almost always fluent and intelligible. Of course, this may not be true of everyone. Grammatical correctness is difficult to assess in a culturally unbiased and practical manner. To evaluate this aspect of verbal interaction you must allow for culturally appropriate language differences, natural use of the vernacular, and sentences that are partially complete expansions of child utterances, etc.

Some disfluency and unintelligibility is to be expected, and adults do not always speak in fully grammatical sentences. However, it is characteristic of child-directed speech to be fluent, intelligible, and grammatical. Chapman (1979) reported only 0.1 percent disfluency, near 100 percent intelligibility, and 60 to 70 percent grammatically correct utterances in studies of mothers' speech to young children. An adult model that has a high degree of disfluency or low intelligibility and grammaticality may indicate a failure to adjust to the child's needs.

Variety of Sentence Types Used. The adult's use of different sentence types allows the child to hear different syntactic structures and to experience different communicative intents. By computing the percentage of questions and imperative and declarative sentences the adult uses, the clinician gains information on the variety of sentences to which the child is exposed.

Procedure and Formula
The computation procedure is the same as that given for other percentages.

Number of utterances that are questions ÷ number of total utterances × 100 = percentage of questions

(Use the same basic formula for each measure.)

Interpretation
Studies have shown that mothers' language to young children includes a large proportion of questions, often as high as 49 percent. Chapman (1979) reported an average of 41.6% questions for six studies of speech to normal, one- to three-year-old children. Although this finding may be an artifact of the way the data were gathered, a similarly high percentage of questions should probably not alarm the evaluator. Chapman (1979) also reported an average of only 14.6 percent imperatives used in the same six studies. A large proportion of imperatives (commands) has been found by some researchers to be more typical of the language used with language-disordered children that with normal language learners (Cross, 1984). Consequently, a high percentage of imperative structures may be cause for concern. The average percentage of declarative sentences for the previously mentioned six studies was 30.5 percent (Chapman, 1979). Declarative sentences (comments) have been found to facilitate language learning (Cross, 1984).

Use

A third important component of the language model is language use in a variety of social situations. One aspect of language use that has been found to be important to language learning is the issue of topic control.

Topic Control: Percentage of Semantically Related and Unrelated Responses. An adult engaged in interaction with a young child can either introduce topics of conversation or respond to topics that the child introduces. If the adult responds (stays on the same topic), he or she may imitate the child's utterance, expand on the utterance by repeating it in a more grammatically complete manner, or elaborate on the same topic with a new utterance that includes some new information. Utterances are considered to be semantically related if they maintain the same topic as the child's last utterance or action. If the adult introduces a new, semantically unrelated topic, he or she initiates conversation about something the child was not previously interested in. Semantically unrelated utterances may also be continuations of an adult-initiated topic or self-repetitions. Computation of the percentage of semantically related and unrelated utterances of the various types gives information on who has control of topic selection in the dyad.

Procedure and Formula

1. Count the total number of adult responses.

2. Go back and count each utterance that is semantically related (or unrelated). Note: semantically related responses could also be broken down into imitations (IM), expansions (EX), and elaborations (EL), and semantically unrelated responses could also be broken down into initiations (IN) and self-repetitions (SR).

3. Divide the number of semantically related (or unrelated) utterances by the total number of utterances and multiply by 100 to find the percent.

Number of semantically (un)related responses ÷ number of total responses × 100 =
percentage of semantically (un)related responses

Interpretation

The adult's use of semantically related responses has been found to be positively related to language ability in children (Cross, 1984; Snow, 1984). A high percentage of unrelated responses should be considered a reason for concern.

Assessing the Consequences of the Child's Communication Attempts

In addition to providing a language model for the language-learning child, family members and others in the child's environment provide feedback for the child's attempts at communication. They accept or reject these attempts and respond in a number of other ways that help to shape the child's attitude toward communication.

To assess the feedback that the child is getting for attempts at communication we can ask several questions:

- Do most of the child's communication attempts get the desired results?
- Are they accepted or rejected?
- Are attempts routinely interrupted so that they cannot be completed?
- Is a response of some kind usually given?

Percentage of Accepting Responses. To assess the consequences of the child's attempts at communication the clinician needs some way to look at the feedback the child is getting on those attempts. One factor to consider is whether the adult's response is one that shows acceptance of the child's attempt. Utterances can be considered to be accepting if they

- are positive or nonevaluative statements about feelings or actions
- seek or convey agreement
- seek or provide information
- praise or encourage the child
- repeat or paraphrase the child's previous utterance

Utterances can be considered nonaccepting if they

- are directive or commanding
- pressure the child to speak or act
- reject the child's idea or action
- express negative evaluation (criticism)
- question information given by the child or indicate a lack of understanding

Procedure and Formula
The computation procedure is the same as that given for other percentages.

Number of accepting utterances ÷ number of total utterances × 100 = percentage of accepting utterances

Interpretation
It is probably neither possible nor desirable to respond to a child in an accepting manner 100 percent of the time. However, at least 75 to 80 percent accepting responses would appear to be helpful to the child who is trying to develop language proficiency. I know of no data on a critical level of accepting responses.

Other Responses to the Child's Communication Attempts. Three other responses to the child's attempts to communicate may be helpful to our understanding of the feedback he or she is getting: (1) percent interruptions, (2) percent of time the adult gives no discernible response (NDR), and (3) percent of the time that the adult provides the goods or services (PDGS) the child requests all give information on the amount of satisfaction or reinforcement the child receives for communication attempts. An utterance is judged to be an interruption if it begins while another speaker is speaking. If the adult gives no verbal or nonverbal indication of having heard the other speaker's utterance, it is considered to be an instance of "no discernible response." If the adult responds to the child by providing the thing or service the child has requested, it is counted as an instance of "provision of desired goods or services."

Procedure and Formula
The computation procedure is the same as that given for other percentages.

Number of interruptions ÷ number of total responses × 100 = percentage of interruptions

(Use the same basic formula for other measures.)

Interpretation
Interpretation of this information must be subjective because little or no research has been done on the effects of these variables on language learning. Common sense dictates that high percentages of interruptions and NDR will have negative effects on language learning, while a high degree of PDGS will have positive effects on motivation to communicate.

Assessing the Time Factors

Time factors are important to both the child's ability to benefit from the language model and the consequences of the child's attempts at communication. Two time-related aspects of the adult language model may be of interest to the clinician. The adult's speech (articulation) rate, measured in syllables per minute (SPM), gives information on the speed at which the language model is presented to the child. This rate is a partial indicator of how much time the child has to process the linguistic message, and of the speed he or she may be trying to imitate. The time between consecutive adult utterances, measured in seconds pause time (SPT), is the time during which the child can finish processing what the adult has said and formulate a response or think of a new topic to initiate. (Percent interruptions can also be considered as a time factor.)

Procedure

A stop watch is required for these measures. A sample of parent utterances (e.g., three one-minute segments) is transcribed and the syllables are counted for each segment of the sample. The utterances are then timed with the stop watch, stopping the watch during any measurable pauses. (I usually exclude single-word utterances because they are difficult to time.) The total number of syllables spoken is then divided by the total speaking time, excluding pauses, resulting in a syllable-per-second rate. Multiply this by 60 to get the syllable-per-minute rate.

For the average number of seconds pause time, identify consecutive adult utterances and time the pauses between these utterances. The total number of seconds divided by the total number of consecutive utterances is the average SPT.

Formulas

Number of total syllables ÷ total speaking time × 60 = SPM
Number of total seconds between utterances ÷ number of total consecutive utterances = SPT

Interpretation

A number of studies have shown that time factors change (the rate gets faster) in normal child-directed speech as the child grows older and that these factors may be important to the auditory perception of the language disordered child (Chapman, 1979; Cross, 1977, 1984). Some studies have also shown that slowing the language model (decreasing SPM and increasing SPT) is associated with speech and language improvement of the child (Guitar et al., 1981, and in press; Kilburg, 1985). A SPM of 230 is considered the upper range of normal, with 196 SPM being the mean (Andrews & Ingham, 1971).

Data from the selected analyses can be recorded on forms such as the one reproduced in Exhibit 6-6. The results of the analyses can then be entered on a record form such as the one in Exhibit 6-7.

CONCLUSION

This discussion of family assessment has suggested a number of ways in which a speech-language pathologist might become involved in helping family members to identify their concerns, priorities, and resources. The next chapter will discuss assessment of the child's communication ability.

Exhibit 6-6 Communication Analysis Form

Name:	Language Model												Consequences				Time			
Date:	Content		Form								Use									
Time: / Utterance #:	Tokens	Types	Here & Now	Morphemes	Disfluencies	Unintelligible	Grammatically Correct	Imperative	Declarative	Question	Semantically Related	Unrelated	Accepting	Interruptions	No Response	Desired Goods & Services	Syllables	Seconds	Pause	

Exhibit 6-7 Summary Sheet

Name: _____ Relationship to Child: _____ Duration of Sample(s): _____

Date(s): _____ Number of Utterances: _____

Measure		Results		Comments
Language Model		**Time 1**	**Time 2**	
Content	TTR			
	% Here and Now			
Form	MLU (Adult)			
	MLU (Child)			
	Difference			
	% Disfluent			
	% Unintelligible			
	% Grammatically Correct			
	% Questions			
	% Imperatives			
	% Declaratives			
Use	% Semantically Related			
	-Imitation			
	-Expansion			
	-Elaboration			
	-Initiation			
	-Self-Repetition			
Consequences				
	% Accepting Responses			
	% Interruptions			
	% No Discernible Response			
	% Provision of Desired Goods and Services			
Time Factors				
	Syllables/Minute			
	Seconds Pause Time			

Appendix 6-A

Clinical Example: Todd and Mrs. C.

A clinical example may be helpful as an illustration of the use of the protocol discussed in this chapter. The following example is adapted from an actual family whose identifying information has been changed.

The child client was a 33-month-old boy who will be called Todd. Todd's mother, who will be called Mrs. C., contacted the clinic to schedule a speech-language evaluation for her son because she had become very concerned about his communication development. She reported that Todd had only recently begun to use one-word utterances and was now "stuttering," especially when he was excited or tired. Observation revealed that most of Todd's attempts at verbal communication were characterized by repetitions of a single syllable, usually "huh" (/h /), accompanied by an exaggerated sentence intonation pattern. These repetitions were sometimes followed by a single morpheme (e.g., "huh-huh-huh-TV"). The behavior that Mrs. C. referred to as stuttering consisted of easy repetitions of the first syllable of words or of whole single-syllable words or nonmeaningful syllables such as "huh." Todd exhibited no apparent anxiety about these repetitions. In most cases, Todd's repetitions appeared more like a form of jargon using a single syllable than stuttering.

An interview with Mrs. C. revealed that she was very concerned about Todd's speech and language development, especially because her older child, a five-year-old daughter named Katie, had been an early talker whose language and speech development had proceeded rapidly. When she compared the two children, something she said she knew she shouldn't do, she often feared that Todd was retarded. Todd's father, who was frequently away from home on business, had not shared her concern, however. Mrs. C. had sought the opinion of her parents-in-law, who made her feel that her concerns were "silly." Mrs. C. reported that she didn't know what to think, but that she continued to feel concerned and couldn't even discuss the issue with her family.

Todd and his mother were seen for three one-hour evaluation sessions at one-week intervals, during the first of which a 20-minute sample of mother-child interaction was videotaped. A portion of the transcript of that sample is presented in Exhibit 6-A-1. Thirty utterances are presented as an illustration. For actual clinical use, a longer sample of at least 50 utterances should be used for greater reliability. This sample was recorded in a clinic playroom that was equipped with a toy sink, a child-sized cabinet/stove, cars, trucks, blocks, a tractor, toy animals, and a toy barn. The mother and child were seated on the floor, playing together, throughout the sample. This segment of the interaction occurred after about six minutes of play.

Using a transcript like this and a videotape of interaction, the clinician can apply any measures from the protocol that seem to be appropriate after the sample is viewed. In this case, all measures in the protocol except percentage of grammatically correct utterances were performed on the mother's utterances. Measures of grammatical correctness were not completed because it did not appear to be a concern for this dyad. Data from the analyses were recorded on the form presented in Exhibit 6-A-2. Exhibit 6-A-3 was used to facilitate the type-token analysis. You may wish to refer to Chapter 6 to review the analysis procedures for each of the measures.

After the data were recorded on the form in Exhibit 6-A-2, calculations for each of the measures were completed and the results were recorded on the form in Exhibit 6-A-4. Each of the results can be considered in turn using the information in the "interpretation" sections for each of the measures discussed in the text.

LANGUAGE MODEL

Content

Type-Token Ratio (TTR). This TTR of 0.41 is well within the limits of what may be considered to be normal. That is, Mrs. C is using vocabulary that is not too diverse for a child who is learning language. She appears to be repeating words often enough for Todd to "tune in" to their referents, at least in this small sample.

Here-and-Now Utterances. All of Mrs. C's utterances have to do with things in the immediate environment, again allowing Todd to link words with their referents.

These two results suggest that the content of Mrs. C's language model should be adequate for Todd to grasp the meaning of words.

Form

Mean Length of Utterance. Mrs. C's average utterance length for this sample is 5.93 morphemes; Todd's is 1.20 morphemes. (Values for a larger sample from the same session were 5.42 morphemes [mother] and 1.40 morphemes

Exhibit 6-A-1 Form for Recording Interaction: Todd and Mrs. C

Child Vocal/Verbal	Child (→) or Adult (←) Nonverbal	Adult Vocal/Verbal
/nom/ [NO]	→ Todd looks at a toy sink-moves toward it.	1. What're you gonna do?
	→ T. Looks at Mother.	2. Where's the other car?
	Mo. picks up cars	3. There's the other car?
		The one with the lady in it.
/m-hm/	→ T. reaches to get car from Mo.'s hand-turns back to sink	4. Can you get that one?
		5. Play your little car game again?
/ha ha/		
	→ Turns toward mo., then back to sink	6. Wanta play your car game again?
	T. continues to face sink	7. Wanta see if you can hit your car with my car?
/no/		
		8. No! ?
(coughs)		
	Mo. plays w/tractor ←	9. I'm gonna put the sheep in this.
(Coughs 3 times)		
	→ T. stays at sink	10. Here
/mhmhm/		
		11. Well what are you gonna do with the sink?
	→ T. continues to look at the sink	12. The sink doesn't work.
		13. Do you have a sink at home?
/hIns ijʌ ha ha ha ha ha ha/		
	Moves tractor looks at Todd ←	14. Tractor's gonna go
	→ T. moves toward mo. & tractor.	15. Wanta see if you can hit your car with the tractor?

Exhibit 6-A-1 Continued

Child Vocal/Verbal	Child (→) or Adult (←) Nonverbal	Adult Vocal/Verbal
Yeah	→ Todd looks at mother moves toward her	
		16. OK, here it goes
		17. There it goes
	→ crashes car w/ truck	
		18. Oh, you're tough! (laughs)
	mo. smiles broadly ←	19. You're a rough guy
		20. You are a rough guy
		21. Yes, you are
	→ crashes toys again	
		22. Todd! (with displeasure)
		23. OK, build them up and then you can knock them down
/hm/		
	mo. pulls blocks closer ←	24. Go on-look at all of 'em
	→ T. manipulates blocks	25. Lots of 'em
/mhm ʌhaa haɪ[high]/		
		26. You gonna build it up high?
/hm ha ha ha/	→ Todd builds small tower /w blocks	
/no no no haɪ[no high]/		
	→ crashes tower	27. No high?
	Mo. smiles weakly ←	28. You can make it higher than that.
	Mo. gestures to blocks ←	29. Make it real high and then you can knock it down
/ba ba bo bo bo bo	→ Todd gestures at blocks looks at Mo.	
ha ha ha ha/		
		30. (Laughs) what does that mean, huh?

Exhibit 6-A-2 Communication Analysis Form for Mrs. C.

Name: Mrs. C   Date: 3/2   Time: 10:00AM

Utterance #	Tokens	Types	Here & Now	Morphemes	Disfluencies	Unintelligible	Grammatically Correct	Imperative	Declarative	Question	Semantically Related	Unrelated	Accepting	Interruptions	No Response	Desired Goods & Services	Syllables	Seconds	Pause
1	5	5	✓	5							✓	IN					6	.47	
2	5	5	✓	5					✓			IN					5		4.41
3	12	6	✓	12						✓		IN					13	5.38	
4	5	3	✓	5					✓			IN					5		
5	6	5	✓	6							✓	IN					8	.91	3.28
6	6	1	✓	6							✓	SR					8	.85	4.13
7	11	4	✓	11					✓			IN					12	1.37	2.35
8	1	1	✓	1					✓			IM					*1		4.66
9	8	5	✓	8						✓		IN	✓				8	.63	3.56
10	1	1	✓	1						✓		IN					*1		4.53
11	9	2	✓	9							✓	IN					10	1.06	5.25
12	4	2	✓	6					✓			IN					5	.81	1.66
13	7	4	✓	7						✓		IN					7	.75	4.56
14	4	2	✓	4					✓			IN	✓				5	3.15	11.94
15	11	0	✓	11						✓		IN					13		
16	4	1	✓	5					✓			IN	✓				5	1.6	2.32
17	3	0	✓	4					✓			IN	✓				3		
18	4	2	✓	4					✓			IN	✓				3		1.71
19	5	2	✓	5					✓			IN	✓				4	7.1	
20	5	0	✓	5					✓			SR	✓				5		
21	3	1	✓	3					✓			IN	✓				3		
22	1	1	✓	1								IN					*1		2.19
23	11	7	✓	11				✓				IN					12	2.0	1.56
24	7	4	✓	7				✓				IN					7	3.86	2.57
25	3	1	✓	4					✓			IN	✓				3		
26	6	1	✓	6						✓		EX	✓				6	.81	6.9
27	2	0	✓	2					✓			IM	✓				2	.40	6.97
28	7	2	✓	7				✓				IN					8	2.72	6.31
29	11	1	✓	11				✓				IN					11		
30	5	2	✓	6						✓		IN					5	1.38	7.38

*NOT COUNTED

Exhibit 6-A-3 Type-Token Ratio Analysis Form

A	B	C	D	E	F
are (what're) again am (I'm) a at and all	build	car can	do (does) doesn't down		

G	H	I	J	K	L
gonna get game go (goes) guy	hit here have home high (higher) huh	is in it if I		knock	lady little look lots

M	N	O	P	Q	R
my make mean	no	other one ok oh or of	play put		rough real

S	T	U	V	W.X	Y.Z
see sheep sink	the then there than that this tractor tough Toda them ('em)	up		what where with wanta well work	you your yes

Exhibit 6-A-4 Summary Sheet for Mrs. C.

Name: **Mrs. C** Relationship to Child: **Mo.** Duration of Sample(s): _____

Date(s): **3/2** Number of Utterances: **30**

Measure		Results		Comments
		Time 1	**Time 2**	
Language Model				
Content	TTR	.41		
	% Here and Now	100%		
Form	MLU (Adult) (178/30)	5.93m.		
	MLU (Child) (6/5)	1.20m.		only intelligible utterances used. MLU for a larger sample was 1.40 morphemes.
	Difference	4.73m.		
	% Disfluent	0		
	% Unintelligible	0		
	% Grammatically Correct	—		
	% Questions	43.3%		
	% Imperatives	10%		
	% Declaratives	43.3%		
Use	% Semantically Related	63.3%		
	-Imitation	10.5% of Sem. Rel.		Todd says little that could be imitated or expanded
	-Expansion	5% of Sem. Rel.		
	-Elaboration	0%		
	-Initiation	90.9% of unrelated		
	-Self-Repetition	9% of Unrel.		
Consequences				
	% Accepting Responses	36.7%		
	% Interruptions	0		
	% No Discernible Response	0		
	% Provision of Desired Goods and Services	0		child made no requests, verbally
Time Factors				
	Syllables/Minutes (182/35.35)	308.9		
	Seconds Pause Time (88.24/29)	3.04		

[Todd].) The difference between these values is 4.73 morphemes. This is a rather large difference compared with the average difference suggested by the literature of about 2.4 morphemes. This may indicate that Mrs. C has not adjusted the length of her utterances to a beneficial length that might give Todd the slightly more complex model that he needs. Her sentences might be too long or complex for him to process readily or to imitate.

Percent Disfluent and Unintelligible. None of Mrs. C's utterances were disfluent or unintelligible. Her model was presented clearly.

Variety of Sentence Types—Questions, Imperatives, Declaratives. The percentage of questions does not exceed the percentage of questions addressed to normal language using children reported in the literature. The percentage of imperatives is likewise not abnormally high. Declaratives are at a reasonable level. It is interesting to note, however, that many of Mrs. C's questions to Todd appear to pressure him to do or pay attention to things that he doesn't seem interested in. Redirecting Todd's attention to something that she chooses may be one way Mrs. C increases her chances of having some idea of what Todd is talking about because his speech is of poor intelligibility. This may be a functional tactic, but it probably doesn't promote language learning.

The form of Mrs. C's utterances appears to be adequate as a language model except in the length/complexity of her sentences. Shorter utterances might be more helpful.

Use

Percentage of Semantically Related Responses. Almost two-thirds (63.3 percent) of Mrs. C's utterances are related to something that Todd is paying attention to. (For a longer sample, only 40.9 percent of Mrs. C's utterances were semantically related.) Still, most of her utterances are initiations, showing that she is often choosing the topic of conversation. This is probably influenced by the fact that Todd uses few intelligible utterances to which she could respond. For this child a higher percentage of semantically related responses might be helpful, with the mother following his lead in both play and verbal interaction. In this sample, Mrs. C failed to attend to the toy that Todd was most interested in (the sink), and attempted instead to get him interested in cars and blocks.

CONSEQUENCES

Percent Accepting Responses. Only 36.7 percent of Mrs. C's utterances in interaction with Todd are accepting in this sample. (In a larger sample, 47.7

percent are accepting.) In other words, almost two-thirds of his mother's utterances to him are nonaccepting. This high proportion of nonacceptance may interfere with his motivation to attempt to communicate. It should be noted that all of Mrs. C's utterances have been analyzed for this measure, not just her responses to Todd's attempts at verbal communication. The result, therefore, is an assessment of the general "tone" of communication that is addressed to him. A more accepting, less pressuring communication environment would probably encourage attempts at verbal communication.

Percent Interruptions, No Discernible Response, Provision of Desired Goods and Services. Mrs. C doesn't interrupt, always responds, and has no opportunity to provide verbally requested goods or services because Todd makes no verbal requests. She fails to respond positively, however, to Todd's nonverbal "request" to play with the sink (see utterances 11 and 12). More accepting responses might encourage more attempts at verbal requests on Todd's part.

TIME FACTORS

Syllables Per Minute and Seconds Pause Time. Mrs. C's articulation rate of 308.9 syllables per minute is well above the upper range of normal (230 SPM) noted in the literature. (Her rate for a longer sample was 350 SPM.) Indeed, it was often difficult to transcribe her speech because it was so fast. Her average pause time between utterances (3.04 seconds) was also very brief. Todd is being presented with a language model that is fast and allows little time between utterances for him to process what has been said and formulate a response or initiate a new topic. One might speculate that his form of jargon-like repetition is an attempt to talk faster and sound more like Mom. A slower model with longer pauses might allow him to have more success in imitating what his mother says (one strategy for language learning), understanding what is said, and participating in the verbal interchange.

In summary this analysis suggests that Todd might benefit from: (1) shorter, less complex, adult utterances; (2) utterances that are semantically related to Todd's play, verbal and nonverbal communication; (3) utterances that are accepting; and (4) utterances delivered more slowly and with longer pauses for Todd to speak.

Appendix 7-C contains further information on Todd's communication abilities at the time of evaluation.

7

Assessment of Child Communication Competence

The primary contribution of the communication specialist to the assessment of very young children is the detailed evaluation of their communication, speech, language, and hearing. This evaluation, and the appropriate treatment that it makes possible, may help to alleviate some of the costs, both monetary and social, of communication disorders. According to Rossetti (1986), early detection and evaluation of developmental delay "improves the outcome for children and families by preventing secondary understimulation or excessive pressure to perform, and it allows for the utilization of existing strengths in the child, the family, and the community" (p. 105).

Unfortunately, developmental problems are seldom identified at or shortly after birth. Palfrey, Singer, Walker, and Butler (1987) conducted a study of 1,726 children in five communities and found that only about 4 percent of disabling conditions were identified at the time of birth. Another 16.4 percent were identified before 3 years of age and 28.7 percent were identified before the age of 5 years; 47.9 percent were identified during early elementary school years and 23.3 percent were detected at 8 years or older. The average age of identification of congenital hearing impairment, for example, is 18 months (Hays, 1989). Better efforts at early identification are needed so that all children and their families can benefit from early preventive intervention.

Communication abilities are complex skills, often built on other behaviors, such as respiratory and motor abilities, which may be overlooked or understressed by other professionals because they are not obviously of paramount importance to the survival of the child. Speech-language pathologists are acutely aware of the importance of infant and toddler communication skills and can share this awareness with the rest of the evaluation team. Communication skills allow the child both to receive important input from the people and

Source: From "The Assessment of Emerging Communication" by G. Donahue-Kilburg, *Communicative Disorders, 7,* pp. 87–101. Portions of this chapter are adapted with permission of Grune and Stratton, Inc., © 1982.

things in the environment and to participate in interactions that contribute to development in general. Assessment of communication skills can help caregivers to engage the child in interactions that are appropriate to his or her abilities. These appropriate interactions can provide the child with important opportunities to improve communication skills. As Seibert, Hogan, and Mundy (1982) have stated, ". . . interventions that provide the caregiver with expanded categories for interpreting the child's signals, modifying how they interact, may give the child more opportunities to acquire and practice missing competencies" (p. 245).

This chapter explores the topic of assessment of communication abilities in infants and toddlers. Its focus is on the child's use of communication within the family context and discusses problems of assessment, the content of the assessment, and methods of communication assessment. It is not an exhaustive treatment of multidisciplinary assessment. For a more thorough discussion of the various areas of assessment other than communication, see Rossetti (1990) or Bailey and Wolery (1989).

Assessment of a very young child's communication, speech, language, and hearing is a demanding process. It entails eliciting, observing, and recording a wide range of behaviors in context, and then interpreting or evaluating those behaviors in relationship to a standard of normal development, taking into consideration the child's and/or family's health status, age, culture, and other individual differences. Rossetti (1986) describes infant assessment as

> . . . any activity either formal (through use of standardized norm referenced criteria) or informal (through use of developmental profiles or checklists) that is designed to elicit accurate and reliable infant behaviors upon which inferences relative to developmental skill status may be made. (p. 101)

It is important to note that assessment activities are not only those formal activities that are designed to test a child's abilities. As Rossetti (1991) stresses, assessment can be any activity. Further, the more instances of infant and toddler behavior which can be observed, the more accurate the assessment of communication will be.

Campbell (1990, April) discriminates between the terms *evaluation* and *assessment.* Citing the distinction drawn in P.L. 99-457, she suggests that evaluation refers to the procedures that establish the child's eligibility for services and that allow for a description of the child's performance. On the other hand, assessment refers to the ongoing process by which professionals identify the child's and family's strengths and needs for services. While this distinction is a useful one within the context of the law, it is not the usual practice in discussions of early intervention. Hutinger (1988), for example, uses the terms in quite the opposite way that Campbell uses them. Because evaluation and assessment generally entail the same kind of data gathering, the terms will be used interchangeably in this chapter.

PURPOSES OF ASSESSMENT

An assessment of a child's communication ability may be done for a number of reasons. It may be done to: (1) track progress and describe normal development; (2) to gauge the impact of medical or environmental factors on an infant or toddler's performance; (3) to detect developmental delay in order to prescribe intervention and check progress during or after intervention; or (4) to determine which children need to be monitored for possible later developmental problems (Rossetti, 1986). The assessment may identify clear disabilities, hidden handicaps, or high-risk situations (Scott & Hogan, 1982).

OBJECTIVES OF ASSESSMENT

The objective of the assessment is not simply to conclude that the abilities are "normal" or "abnormal," or to provide all-too-obvious "diagnoses." The process must yield detailed descriptive information on the characteristics and frequency of the communication skills used by the child, the age appropriateness of the skills, the physical and/or cognitive appropriateness of the skills, the "goodness of fit" of the skills with environmental conditions and requirements, and information on how to enhance and support communication strengths and improve areas of weakness. It may also give information on possible factors that

The test results are in and it seems you have a growth on your knee, Mr. Smith.

contribute to the etiology and/or maintenance of a communication disorder as well as existing factors that can facilitate communication growth.

ISSUES AND PROBLEMS OF EARLY ASSESSMENT

There are a number of assumptions that underlie early assessment efforts. Professionals often assume that development occurs in a predictable manner and that all normal children follow a given course of development. If we think that development is continuous and that early experience and ability foretell later performance, we may also assume that early assessment has some predictive value. Unfortunately, tests of early ability, especially those administered in infancy, have been found to have little predictive validity (Anastasi, 1982). This may be because the sample of behavior obtained for the test is not a reliable sample (Rossetti, 1991), because the items the tests contain do not adequately tap the skills that are continuous with later abilities, or because many early and later abilities are, in fact, not continuous. Sameroff (1975) suggests the possibility that ". . . linear sequences are non-existent and that development proceeds through a sequence of regular restructurings of relations within and between the organism and his environment" (p. 285). If this is the case, measures can only be expected to assess current abilities; there is no foolproof way to assess how the organism will be "restructured" at a future time.

The lack of predictive value of most early assessment tools should not be seen as evidence that early assessment is futile, however. While a single administration of a single test may not predict the future, infant assessment does give information on the child's current abilities that can be used to prescribe current treatment. Further, multiple or serial assessments, made at different times and/or using different methods, increase the reliability of the information gathered and the validity of our predictive statements as well as the value of our current assessment (Rossetti, 1986; Sparks, 1989). As Kagan (1971) pointed out, infant responses are like windows of a house, each window gives a different glimpse of the contents and structure of the house. To get a coherent picture of the interior, however, you must have many points of view—many windows to look through. Rossetti (1986) has summarized these issues well:

> The best possible way in which the practitioner can view assessment results is as an indicator of the child's performance on the day the testing was performed, not as an indicator of future potential for developmental skill acquisition. Oftentimes the word diagnosis is applied to infant assessment. The use of this word is best left in the medical model because a medical diagnosis leads to definitive statements about etiology, clinical symptomatology, treatment, and prognosis. Educational or psychological testing provides little or no information about etiology, some but not much about clinical symptomatology, and absolutely none about prognosis. A single testing can be viewed as only a glimpse into child behavior on a particular day and under a particular set of circumstances. (p. 106)

In addition to the problem of prediction of later outcome from early assessment, there are some special problems related to the process of assessing young children. There are several areas that are important for clinicians to consider when assessing very young children: the test situation, the child's physical state, response repertoire, ability to attend to adult-selected stimuli, tendency toward distractibility, level of psychosocial development, and degree of socialization. Each of these problems will be discussed in light of its impact on these and other aspects of the traditional assessment situation and formal test administration.

Test Situation

The physical test situation that is prescribed by most traditional, formal language tests is a "clinical" situation. It is usually suggested that this setting should have few stimuli other than a table at which the child and examiner are seated. This arrangement is quite different from the typical infant's or toddler's accustomed environment. In the child's experience, it is probably most like the physician's office, which is not necessarily a pleasant association. In addition, it is sometimes recommended by the test developer that the child's parents or caregivers be excluded from this test situation so that they will not answer for the child, unwittingly give clues, or in some other way confound the child's responses.

In reality, the situations in which clinicians often find themselves attempting to assess young children are very different from those prescribed by these tests. When we assess children in their own homes, the environment is sometimes chaotic with other children, a loud television or radio, pets, cramped conditions, etc., all contributing their own stimuli. When we work in some institutional settings there may be similar problems. For example, some day care settings have little room for quiet, controlled presentation of test items. Arena assessments, described in Chapter 4, are often a good way to observe the infant or toddler responding to a variety of stimuli, but may not allow for the completion of a detailed test protocol if several professionals have items to be administered.

Physical State

The infant's or toddler's physical state deserves some attention in relationship to assessment of communication behaviors. The infant's state of alertness as described by Brazelton (1983) is an important consideration in determining the infant's ability to participate at an optimal level in the observation or evaluation of his or her communication behavior. Rossetti (1990) defines infant state as ". . . the level of alertness and environmental interaction patterns present in an infant or toddler at a given point" (p. 106). Brazelton (1983) labels and defines these states as follows:

Sleep states

1. Deep sleep with regular breathing, eyes closed, no spontaneous activity except startles or jerky movements at quite regular intervals; . . .

2. Light sleep with eyes closed; rapid eye movements can often be observed under closed lids; low activity level. . . . Respirations are irregular, sucking movements occur off and on. Eye opening may occur briefly at intervals.

Awake states

3. Drowsy or semi-dozing; eyes may be open but dull and heavy-lidded, or closed, eyelids fluttering; activity level variable. . . . Dazed look when the infant is not processing information and is not "available."

4. Alert, with bright look; seems to focus invested attention on source of stimulation. . . . Motor activity is at a minimum. There is a kind of glazed look which can be easily broken through in this state.

5. Eyes open; considerable motor activity, with thrusting movements of the extremities . . . reactive to external stimulation. . . . Brief fussy vocalizations occur in this state.

6. Crying; characterized by intense crying which is difficult to break through with stimulation; motor activity is high. (p. 18)

An infant who is in anything but state 4, which is often called the quiet alert state, will not respond optimally to environmental stimuli. Because it is difficult to influence the infant's state, it is wise to plan the assessment for the time when the infant is most likely to be in a quiet alert state (e.g., after nap time) or to allow for flexible timing of evaluations (e.g., by planning a lengthy visit with other objectives such as a parent interview which might be accomplished while waiting for the infant to wake up or eat) to accommodate different states.

With infants and toddlers who are not yet able to verbalize their needs and complaints, unknown factors related to their physical condition may greatly influence their state of alertness and comfort and therefore their test performance. Children may be tired or hungry, may have undiagnosed otitis media, or a host of other covert physical factors may operate to depress their ability to perform at their optimal level. Communicative ability seems to be one of the first behaviors to suffer from the effects of such physical factors. The young child often responds to fatigue, hunger, and illness by crying, a behavior which precludes use of the vocal tract for higher-level symbolic function. Unless the physical difficulty that the child is experiencing can be dealt with in the clinical situation (e.g., feeding a hungry child), it is often necessary to reschedule the evaluation for a later date.

Response Repertoire

The infant's and toddler's response repertoire is naturally limited by maturation and level of development. For example, six-month-old children's neuromotor systems would not allow for a specific pointing response even if they knew the correct response for an instruction like, "Show me dog."

Language tests require a variety of responses from the child. The ten most common of these responses are presented in Table 7-1. Table 7-1 also includes examples of item stimuli and information concerning the age at which a normal child first can be expected to respond reliably to that kind of item.

The responses in Table 7-1 require a number of different behaviors from the child. Each test may be viewed in terms of the response demands that it places

---

Table 7-1 Responses Commonly Required on Language Tests

Response	Example	Estimate of Youngest Appropriate Age
1. Production of an evoked or spontaneous sample of communicative behavior		6 months or younger
2. Behavioral compliance with commands	"Give me the cup."	12 months
3. Immediate imitation of a spoken stimulus	"Say, 'I saw a big dog.' "	18 months (1 word) 36 months (sentence)
4. Pointing to or "showing" an object or picture named or described by the examiner	a. "Point to dog." (1 word) b. "Show me 'The boy is walking.' " (sentence)	18 months 24–30 months
5. Verbal or gestural response to questions	"Where is your foot?"	20 months
6. Manipulating objects or acting out a sentence	"Put the block on the chair."	20 months
7. Completion of a carrier phrase	"Here is a cat; here are two____."	36 months
8. Paraphrasing a story		36 months
9. Delayed imitation of a spoken stimulus	" 'The baby is crying, the baby is not crying,' now, what's this picture?"	40–48 months
10. Making a judgment about which word or sentence is correct or goes with a stimulus	"Which is right, 'The childs played,' or 'The children played,'?"	42–48 months

on the child. If it requires a heavy concentration of responses with which a given child has difficulty, the results will not be accurate. An obvious problem occurs when a test that requires many pointing responses is used to assess a child with motor deficits in the upper extremities. A less obvious problem occurs when a test that has many items requiring behavioral compliance with commands is used with a two-year-old child who is displaying age-appropriate difficulty with external controls. The most common response of these toddlers to items like "Give me the ball," is "No." Unless the test developer has provided special rules for scoring this kind of response clinicians are assessing tractability rather than communication ability.

Attending Abilities

Traditional language tests require that the person being tested be able to sit down and pay attention for varying periods of time. Even normal infants, of course, are not capable of this behavior for any length of time, and toddlers are often less than cooperative. The ability to attend to a given task develops and improves with age just as other cognitively based abilities do. The very young infant gives only a crude, nonselective, orienting response to external stimuli (Berry, 1969). At first, infants primarily attend to internal stimuli in their own bodies. Attention gradually turns outward, with the infant being able to choose an examiner-presented object to attend to between 9 and 12 months of age (Knobloch & Pasamanick, 1974). When children begin to walk, their attention shifts rapidly in response to almost any external stimulus. This rapid and diverse shifting of attention continues through at least 18 months of age (Knobloch & Pasamanick, 1974). After two years of age, as development continues, children progress from giving fixed attention to a concrete task of their own choice, through allowing an adult to direct their attention, to following adult directions while completing a task (Swope & Liebergott, 1977). Many tests, even those designed for use with young children, require performance at this highest level of attention for about 30 minutes at a time. This is clearly beyond the endurance of most normal children under 36 months of age.

Related to the young child's attending abilities is the problem of distractibility. Extraneous stimuli in the environment are often blamed for poor test performance in children of this age. Some tests designed for use with young children have attractive toy stimuli for use with specific test items. Some tests fail to provide a kit that adequately organizes these stimuli to keep them out of the child's sight. Even in an otherwise bare room, it often becomes difficult for the examiner to handle these stimuli so that they are unseen before and after administration of the given item. Thus, the test stimuli themselves become distracting environmental factors.

In addition to these issues, which relate to both children who are developing normally and who have problems with development, is the special case of prenatally drug-exposed infants. Babies who have been exposed to alcohol may display a variety of symptoms including growth deficiencies, minor physical anomalies such as slightly deformed facial features, and dysfunctions of the central nervous system including mental retardation. Infants who have been exposed to drugs, such as cocaine or heroine, may be lethargic, hypertonic, irritable, jittery, and fail to interact normally or be easily overstimulated (Rossetti, 1990; Kaplan-Sanoff, Parker, & Zuckerman, 1991). These conditions may adversely affect attending abilities.

Level of Psychosocial Development

The clinical setting prescribed for administration of many tests may also create special problems related to the child's level of psychosocial development. Children are thought to go through a process of separation/individuation (see Chapter 2). Through this developmental process, children become aware of themselves in relationship to other people in their environments. For normally developing children, the result of separation/individuation is a healthy awareness of themselves as individuals and an ability to mentally represent and relate to trusted caregivers. At times during this process, children experience periods of acute stranger anxiety and fearful awareness of new and different environments. While this anxiety is a normal by-product of children's increasing awareness of their surroundings, it may often make it difficult to obtain desired responses from young children who are anxious and fearful when introduced to an unfamiliar clinical setting and/or examiner.

It is sometimes recommended by the test developer that the child's parents or caregivers be excluded from the test situation. This recommendation is made for the good reason that it is sometimes difficult for interested and concerned parents to observe passively while their child is evaluated. This is especially true if the evaluation procedures and goals are not carefully explained to the parents. Again, a characteristic of the very young child may make exclusion of the caregiver or parent difficult. Children between birth and three years of age often become upset when separated from the primary caregiver. This condition is sometimes referred to as separation anxiety and is especially likely to occur when the child is placed in an unfamiliar setting and left with a less-than-well-known examiner.

Another factor that must be considered in relationship to the assessment of young children's abilities is their level of socialization. Very young children are poorly socialized. They have not yet internalized the value system which dictates that it is desirable to do what adults want you to do (Anastasi, 1982). Well-socialized five-year-old children may attempt boring tasks just because the examiner asks them to do so, but two-year-old children are not as likely to comply. This can make items requiring behavioral compliance virtually meaningless. It is often impossible to know whether children fail to comply with requests because they do not understand the requests or because they do not wish to comply.

CONTENT OF THE ASSESSMENT: AREAS TO BE ASSESSED

While there are many issues to be decided concerning the assessment of communication in very young children, such as who should be involved in the assessment and where the assessment should take place, no question is more important than what should be assessed. This issue must be decided in order to plan a thorough assessment and to evaluate measurement tools that might be used in that assessment. Broadly, the emphasis of the speech-language pathologist's assessment will be on communication, with attention to both its nonverbal and verbal aspects and emphasis on hearing, oral motor abilities, language, and speech.

The ASHA Committee on Language Subcommittee on Speech-Language Pathology Service Delivery with Infants and Toddlers (1989) suggests that intervention must be based on

> . . . a clinical analysis of a child's mastery or potential for mastery of oral-motor skills as well as the content (knowledge base), form (oral and other symbolic modes of communication), and functions (socio-communicative interaction) required for language and communication. A clinical analysis also must include an assessment of preverbal behaviors that are necessary for the development of adequate communication, language, and speech skills. (p. 33)

More detailed information on the content of an assessment of child communicative competence comes from a study by Kilburg (1980). Kilburg conducted a dual-focused study to establish a content domain to use in the assessment of the content validity of various measures of early communication. First, information concerning important infant-toddler communication behaviors was gathered from experienced clinicians and researchers who worked with infants and toddlers. Then, the content of test items from 12 language tests designed for use with 6- to 36-month-old children was analyzed. Content of the test items was found to fit into ten categories that were similar to those from the clinicians'/researchers' responses.

The content categories from both sources were then combined to form one set of 14 content categories. These categories are listed below, roughly rank ordered according to percentage of items or responses that addressed each one. The definition that is presented with each category includes aspects of the behavior noted by the respondents or covered by the test items, not a thorough definition of the behavior or content area.

1. *Understanding and use of meaningful words.* This category includes behaviors such as responding to simple commands, to one's name, specific words, and measures of vocabulary size.
2. *Nonverbal communication behaviors.* Behaviors classified under this heading include: eye contact, smiling, facial gestures, general affect, gesture, touch, vocalization, laughter, and vocal inflection in both receptive and expressive modes.
3. *Syntax.* Word combinations of four or more words and use of grammatical morphemes are included in this category.
4. *Phonological development.* Includes behaviors such as crying, babbling, producing jargon and specific phonemes, and degree of intelligibility of speech.
5. *Word combinations.* The ability to combine two or three words in an utterance comprises this category. These combinations may be viewed in terms of functions or semantic relations and rules.
6. *Conceptual information.* The child's knowledge of basic concepts, such as colors and size, and ability to categorize items were included here.
7. *Cognitive abilities.* This category includes the ability to imitate, to attend to given stimuli, evidence of object constancy, and other intellectual functioning.
8. *Responses to auditory stimuli.* This category covers information related to the child's reaction to speech or environmental sounds. Responses include alerting, localization, and discrimination.
9. *Pragmatics.* The child's variety of language functions, ability to initiate verbal interaction, and general discourse skills are components of this category.
10. *Play behaviors.* Symbolic, functional, interactive, imaginative, explorative, and stereotyped play as well as the absence of play are among the important categories of play behavior to be observed.
11. *Evidence of oral motor integrity.* This category pertains to feeding behavior, oral motor movements, and muscle tone.
12. *Parent-child interaction.* Behaviors in this category include parent-child verbal interaction and parent's response to the child's communication.
13. *Verbal response to questions.* The ability to give accurate verbal responses to questions comprised this category.

14. *Auditory memory.* Items concerned with memory of digits, words, sentences, etc., are classified here.

Two more content areas, infant state and respiration, may be especially important in the assessment of neonates. Infant state is important to consider before making any other assessments of neonatal behavior. Respiration, which provides the energy for sound making as well as the foundation for physiological stability in general, is another significant aspect of the child's behavior to be considered.

The assessment should also consider the "goodness of fit" of the child's communication skills within the communicative environment (see Chapter 6).

The list of 17 content categories for intant-toddler communication assessment covers a wide range of abilities (see Exhibit 7-1). The categories are not necessarily of equal importance, and their order of presentation is not necessarily indicative of their importance to the development of communication. The list does seem to be useful as a basis for evaluating the content validity of measures of early communication and as a guide to possible assessment content.

METHODS OF ASSESSMENT

Providing assessment services for infants, toddlers, and their families requires some rethinking of traditional approaches to assessment. Most tradi-

---

Exhibit 7-1 List of Content Categories for Infant-Toddler Communication Assessment

 1. Infant state
 2. Respiration
 3. Response to auditory stimuli
 4. Nonverbal communication behaviors
 5. Parent-child interaction
 6. Play behaviors
 7. Understanding and use of meaningful words
 8. Phonological development
 9. Word combinations
10. Syntax
11. Pragmatics
12. Verbal response to questions
13. Auditory memory
14. Conceptual information
15. Evidence of oral motor integrity
16. Cognitive abilities
17. "Goodness of fit" with the communicative environment

tional measures of language ability have been developed to assess school-aged children and have been designed, in keeping with psychometric standards, to sample language behavior, much as a classroom test samples a student's knowledge of given subject matter. These measures take a number of different forms. Standardized norm-referenced measures are designed to compare one child's performance to the "normal" performance of a large, supposedly representative sample of peers. Nonstandardized measures are generally more flexible than standardized procedures, but they do not provide norms of performance for comparison. Developmental scales sample major achievements across an age period to determine the developmental age level of a child. Criterion-referenced measures are designed to assess mastery of a given task, rather than to compare a child's performance to a norm.

For all of these measures, the test developer has made the assumption that a representative sample of language behavior can be obtained in a short period of time, in a "clinical" setting in which little real communication may be taking place. This may or may not be true of school-aged children; it is seldom true of infants and toddlers.

Research and common sense tell us that emerging communication can be viewed accurately only in developmental and environmental contexts. Consequently, clinicians cannot restrict their views to isolated communicative behaviors that can be elicited in a clinical setting. Clinicians must consider a range of cognitive, social, motor, and play behaviors, as well as caregiver and environmental factors, in order to understand how the child communicates. Unfortunately, few commercially available tests are designed to look at all of these variables.

Because of the limitations of most formal assessment tools, especially for use with young children, a trend toward informal assessment began in the 1970s. Informal measures that have been used to fill this need include analysis of spontaneous behavior (language samples and play observations) and a variety of nonstandardized measures that clinicians have devised to fit their own needs. Some approaches to informal assessment are presented later in this chapter.

EVALUATION OF ASSESSMENT TOOLS

Even though there are problems with many of the formal assessment tools designed for use in communication assessment of very young children, it is often necessary to use such a tool to satisfy bureaucratic requirements. It is possible to do this without succumbing to the problems associated with formal measures. One way a clinician can increase the quality of the assessment that is provided for infants and toddlers is to critically evaluate any measure that is considered for use, to use only the best of these measures, and to go beyond the formal measures.

Guidelines for Judging Test Adequacy

To provide a structure for the evaluation of assessment tools, I have devised a form that presents several different areas of evaluation. The form is designed to structure the clinician's review of the measure, not to dictate what a measure "should" include. This evaluation format covers the four major characteristics of a standardized test: (1) conditions for administration, (2) rules for scoring, (3) normative information for interpretation, and (4) procedures for systematic sampling (Mitchell, undated). Because of this emphasis, some sections of the form are probably most useful in evaluating standardized, norm-referenced tests. The sections on materials, content, reliability, and validity, however, are appropriate for any measure. A copy of the evaluation form is presented in Appendix 7-A.

SUGGESTIONS FOR A THOROUGH ASSESSMENT

No test or informal assessment technique is adequate as a thorough assessment tool in itself. Carefully evaluating and combining approaches is the best way to structure an assessment battery. This process can follow some of the suggestions given here, but it is always an individualized process which must be tailored to meet the needs of each child and family. It is important to plan the assessment of the child with input from the parents or other caregivers concerning family preferences for involvement, ideas for time and place of evaluation, and the kinds of information they would especially like to gain from the assessment (Turnbull, 1991). One workable assessment progression is as follows:

1. Before contact, obtain developmental information and history from caregivers and other agencies, and talk with the caregivers about the evaluation so that they will know what to expect and can give their input concerning the best time and place, etc.

2. On initial contact, conduct a parent/caregiver interview to obtain any additional background information. Observe and record (preferably on videotape) parent-child interaction. If this is done in the center, I often suggest to the caregivers that they help their child to feel more comfortable in the new environment by allowing the child to play with the toys, and that they talk with the child as they normally would at home. Play and/or interact with the child yourself after the parent-child interaction, to get a sense of what the child is like to be with. Videotape as much of this first session as possible. Give the parent an at-home assessment questionnaire such as one of the ones listed under "Informal Assessment Strategies." Observe and record in the home if possible.

3. Between sessions, analyze the informal sample of parent-child interaction, looking at both parent and child behaviors (e.g., child's nonverbal and verbal communicative behaviors, the parent's interactive behaviors as language-learning stimuli, and responses as outlined in Chapter 6). Decide on the formal measures to be used with the child and family.

4. During the second and third sessions, do formal testing, specific informal assessment procedures, hearing screening (done free field in the audiology suite, if possible), and obtain another sample of parent-child interaction and child communication behaviors.

INFORMAL ASSESSMENT STRATEGIES

Techniques for informal assessment of child communication have received increasing attention because clinicians and researchers have been dissatisfied with the available formal assessment tools (e.g., Leonard, Prutting, Perozzi, & Berkley, 1978). Even when formal tools are more or less adequate measures of some aspects of early communication, informal strategies are useful as supplemental measures. Informal techniques can certainly be helpful in filling in gaps left by formal measures, and in obtaining information which is difficult to measure by formal methods.

Informal techniques can be especially useful for the following kinds of information:

1. Sampling communication behaviors in context (e.g., in interaction with a caregiver or other family member).

2. Gathering detailed information on behaviors that have been suggested as areas of concern by caregivers, other referral sources, screenings, or the developmental history.

3. Gathering information on the child's communication and related behaviors in his/her usual environment (home or institution). Questionnaires such as Oliver (MacDonald, 1978) and the Infant Communication Questionnaire (Ylvisaker, 1981) may prove helpful in this area if you can't visit the home.

4. Obtaining information on areas not covered well on the formal tests which you use. If you have evaluated your chosen measure using the format presented in Appendix 7-A, you can see which of the suggested content areas are not assessed adequately. You may wish to informally evaluate those areas.

Any of the content areas can be informally assessed. The most important of these may be oral motor ability, parent-child interaction, play, and pragmatics because they are often inadequately addressed by formal tools.

Oral motor skills are especially difficult to assess by standard means in young children. Speech-language pathologists should be specifically trained to use most evaluation procedures such as the Pre-Speech Assessment Scale (Morris, 1982). Informal assessment of oral skills may be done by observing the child while he or she eats and drinks foods of various textures and by asking caregivers to report on the kinds of foods eaten at home and the length of time required for each meal. Conditions related to normal function and abnormal or compensatory oral movement such as those discussed by Jaffe (1989) (see Exhibit 7-2) and by Alexander (1987) can be specifically noted. With older

Exhibit 7-2 Major Movement Patterns Related to Feeding

Primitive Patterns (Usually Seen During the First 6 Months of Infant Development)	Higher Developmental Patterns (Usually Seen Between 6 and 24 Months)	Abnormal and Compensatory Patterns
Suckling: The early infantile method of sucking that involves extension-retraction of the tongue, up-and-down jaw excursions, and low approximations of the lips.	*Munching:* The earliest form of chewing that involves a flattening and spreading of the tongue combined with up-and-down jaw movement.	*Tongue thrust:* An abnormally forceful protrusion of the tongue from the mouth.
Sucking: Characterized by negative pressure in the oral cavity, rhythmic up-and-down jaw movements, tongue tip elevation, firm approximation of the lips, and minimal jaw excursions.	*Chewing:* Characterized by spreading and rolling movements of the tongue propelling foods between the teeth, tongue lateralization, and rotary jaw movements.	*Tongue retraction:* A strong pulling back of the tongue to the pharyngeal space. *Jaw thrust:* An abnormally forceful and tense downward extension of the mandible.
Rooting reaction: Head turning in response to tactile stimulation applied to the lips or around the mouth.	*Tongue lateralization:* Movement of the tongue to the sides of the mouth to propel food between the teeth for chewing.	*Lip retraction:* Drawing back of the lips so that they form a tight line over the mouth. *Lip pursing:* A tight pursestring movement of the lips.
Phasic bite reflex: A rhythmic bite and release pattern, seen as a series of small jaw openings and closings when the teeth or gums are stimulated.	*Rotary jaw movements:* The smooth interaction and integration of vertical, lateral, diagonal, and eventually circular movements of the jaw used in chewing.	*Tonic bite reflex:* An abnormally strong jaw closure when the teeth or gums are stimulated. *Jaw clenching:* An abnormally tight closure of the mouth.
	Controlled, sustained bite: An easy, gradual closure of the teeth on the food, with an easy release of the food for chewing.	

Source: From "Feeding At-Risk Infants and Toddlers" by M. Jaffe, 1989, *Topics in Language Disorders, 10,* p. 15. Copyright 1989 by Aspen Publishers, Inc.

toddlers, various forms of play, such as blowing bubbles, may lead to happy cooperation in oral motor imitation and inspection. If an oral motor, feeding, or swallowing problem appears to exist and you are not trained in detailed assessment of this aspect of behavior, refer the child for a thorough evaluation.

The child's use of communication behaviors, parent-child interaction, and play may often be sampled in one or more observations of the child and caregiver(s) or other family members at play in the home or center. This interaction may be tape recorded while detailed observation notes are made or, preferably, videotaped and analyzed to obtain information on nonverbal communication, play behaviors, vocalization, language function, interactive style, initiation of communicative interchange, turn-taking, word use, various measures of semantic and syntactic ability (e.g., semantic relations, grammatical morphemes, MLU, TTR), or any other child or caregiver behavior which is of interest. See Miller (1981) or Stickler (1987) for specific information on these and other measures. Also see Chapter 6 of this book for methods of analyzing parent communication behaviors.

Roth and Spekman (1984) give useful suggestions for assessing pragmatic abilities, and Wetherby, Yonclas, and Bryan (1989) provide excellent ideas for communication sampling and interpretation of results for young children. Play, as it relates to language, may be informally evaluated using procedures such as those suggested by Westby (1980) or used as the basis for the entire assessment as suggested by Linder (1990).

Another consideration in planning the informal assessment is the context in which behaviors will be sampled. Some factors include

1. the people to be involved: family members, other caregivers, other professionals, aides, students, other children
2. the environment in which the sample will be obtained: clinic, playroom, home, school, or institution
3. the verbal stimuli to be used with the child: giving commands and asking many questions may decrease spontaneous communication, commenting, reflecting, and expanding utterances may increase spontaneous output
4. the other stimuli to be used in the assessment context: pictures, toys, food, situations, play rituals, or games. Wetherby et al. (1989) give an interesting list of conditions that are designed to entice children to initiate communication. These "communicative temptations" include suggestions such as

   — eat a desired food item in front of the child without offering any to the child

   — activate a wind-up toy, let it deactivate, and hand it to the child

   — open a jar of bubbles, blow bubbles, then close the jar tightly; hand the closed jar to the child

— hold a food item or toy that the child dislikes out near the child to offer it (pp. 242-243)

SOME AVAILABLE ASSESSMENT TOOLS

The list of assessment tools that are designed to evaluate infant and toddler communication is growing rapidly. Some tools are measures of general development with a section on communication; others are completely devoted to the assessment of communication abilities. The annotated list which follows presents a selection of the available measures. Tests presented here all screen or assess communication in detail or are otherwise notably useful for assessment. The presence of a measure on this list in no way implies the author's endorsement of its quality. Each measure should be evaluated by the user for the specific population with which it will be used.

Battelle Developmental Inventory.
Authors: J. Guidubaldi, J. Newborg, J. Stock, J. Svinicki, and L. Wnek
Publisher: DLM Teaching Resources, Allen, TX
Date: 1984
Age range: Birth to 8 years
Content: Personal-social, adaptive, motor, communication, and cognition. The *Battelle* is a standardized, norm-referenced measure with both a screening test and a full battery.

Communication Evaluation Chart from Infancy to Five Years.
Authors: R. Anderson, M. Miles, and P. Matheny
Publisher: Educators Publishing Service, Cambridge, MA
Date: 1963
Age range: 3 months to 5 years
Content: Covers a wide range of behaviors in a nonstandardized checklist format, using observation and parent report.

Communication and Symbolic Behavior Scales (Research Edition).
Authors: A. Wetherby and B. Prizant
Publisher: Riverside Press, Chicago, IL
Date: 1992
Age range: Functional communication age 9 months to 2 years
Content: Communication, social, affective, and symbolic abilities. This test is standardized and norms have been developed. Testing is videotaped for later analysis.

Early Language Milestone Scale.
Author: J. Coplan
Publisher: Modern Education Corporation, Tulsa, OK
Date: 1987
Age range: Birth to 3 years
Content: Norm-referenced screening tool for auditory reception, expression, and vision. Designed for use in a physician's office.

Environmental Language Program Diagnostic Components: Environmental Prelanguage Battery (EPB) and **Environmental Language Inventory** (ELI).
Authors: J. MacDonald and D. Horstmeier
Publisher: Charles E. Merrill Publishing Co., Columbus, OH
Date: 1978
Age range: EPB—At or below single-word level
             ELI—First word combinations to four-word sentences
Content: Criterion-referenced measures for describing or prescribing prelanguage and early verbal behaviors (EPB) and semantic relations (ELI).

Infant Scale of Communicative Intent.
Authors: G. Sacks and E. Young
Publisher: St. Christopher's Hospital for Children, Philadelphia, PA
Date: 1982
Age range: Birth to 18 months
Content: Nonstandardized checklist of communication comprehension and expression for describing early abilities based on observation, testing, and parent report.

Pre-Speech Assessment Scale.
Author: S.E. Morris
Publisher: Preston, Clifton, NJ
Date: 1982
Age range: Not specified
Content: Feeding, oral motor, respiration, and phonation rating scale.

MacArthur Communicative Development Inventory: Infants/Toddlers.
Author: Center for Research in Language
Publisher: Center for Research in Language, San Diego, CA
Date: 1990
Age range: Infants and toddlers
Content: Parent report of understanding and production of phrases and vocabulary, games, play, and early syntax. Norms being developed.

Receptive Expressive Emergent Language Scale (2nd Edition).
Authors: K. Bzoch and R. League
Publisher: Pro-Ed, Austin, TX
Date: 1991
Age range: Birth to 3 years
Content: Parent report, developmental scale samples a broad range of language-related behaviors.

Reynell Developmental Language Scales (U.S. Edition).
Authors: J. Reynell and C. Gruber
Publisher: Western Psychological Services, Los Angeles, CA
Date: 1990
Age range: 1 to 6 years
Content: Standardized, norm-referenced assessment of semantic and syntactic development.

The Rossetti Infant-Toddler Language Scale.
Author: L. Rossetti
Publisher: LinguiSystems, East Moline, IL
Date: 1990
Age range: Birth to 36 months
Content: Criterion-referenced assessment of interaction and attachment, gestures, pragmatics, play, and language comprehension and expression.

Sequenced Inventory of Communication Development—Revised.
Authors: D. Hedrick, E. Prather, and A. Tobin
Publisher: Western Psychological Services, Los Angeles, CA
Date: 1984
Age range: 4 months to 4 years
Content: Standardized, norm-referenced test of receptive and expressive communication.

Increasing Information from Standardized Tests

If test norms are to be used to interpret test results, the measure must be administered in a standardized manner. A number of beneficial changes, however, may be made in the organization and presentation of the test without violating its standardization. As noted earlier, test stimuli may become environmental distractions for the child if they are displayed in an open test kit or if they must be "shuffled" excessively during testing. When this occurs, it is necessary to reorganize the test materials to make assessment more efficient and, when possible, less directive. The following suggestions may be helpful.

- Obtain duplicates of any stimuli that are used for more than one test item. This saves reorganization of materials during testing.
- Make a test kit that organizes the materials for easy access and keeps them hidden from the child. My favorite "kit" is a long, loose-fitting jacket on which has been sewn approximately 12 pockets of various sizes. Into each pocket the stimuli for one test item is put. The pocket keeps the stimuli out of sight and close to me until they are introduced. Once the contents of some of the pockets are known to the child, attention often becomes riveted to the jacket and examiner, awaiting further revelations.
- If possible, allow the children to choose the test materials that interest them some of the time. This is possible on some tests that allow flexibility in the order of item presentation if the test items are rearranged according to the stimuli needed for administration. For example, a child could be allowed to choose between such test stimuli as toy cars or colored blocks. Once the choice is made, the examiner could administer all age-appropriate items that use the chosen toys as stimuli. This format helps to decrease the demand that the children constantly redirect their attention to adult-chosen stimuli.

Test scores are useful and sometimes necessary, but they are not the only results from the careful administration of a reasonably good test. It may be necessary to go beyond the test requirements to get a more accurate picture of the child's ability. For example, if scoring standards allow only one presentation of verbal stimuli, only the child's response to that first presentation of the stimulus can be scored. Repetition of the stimulus, however, may often get a different response and give the examiner additional information that can be used in describing the child's abilities in the report and in planning treatment.

It is also possible to look at the quality and quantity of the child's responses to the test items and other incidental interactions during the assessment session. Even incorrect responses should be carefully considered. Why was the response incorrect? Was it a random choice or a confusion within a category? A pattern of errors may become evident and that pattern can help the clinician to understand the specific characteristics of communication difficulty and to plan treatment.

ORGANIZING AND INTERPRETING THE INFORMATION

Appendix 7-B illustrates one possible format for organizing the information from the formal and informal assessment. This form suggests a reorganization of the information from the suggested content areas into an outline of categories from which a report could be written. The far right-hand column on the form can be used to record evaluative comments or normative information from developmental charts.

Once the information has been organized, the child's abilities can be thoroughly described and areas of proficiency and deficiency can be noted. The clinician may also conjecture concerning possible causal factors related to deficiencies that may have common cognitive, physical, or environmental roots or prerequisite behaviors. Appendix 7-C contains a case illustration using the form.

If the child who has been assessed was born prematurely, an additional consideration must be made. A correction for prematurity should be made in test results for at least one year after birth (Rossetti, 1986, 1991) unless, with repeated testing, the child displays catch-up growth (age-appropriate behavior). According to Rossetti (1986), ". . . if an infant displays a developmental delay on early test administration but subsequently displays rapid catch-up growth with no delay present by 12 to 15 months of age (no need to correct for prematurity), a more favorable prognosis is possible" (p. 135). In fact, Rossetti (1991) suggests that catch-up growth may be the best barometer for predicting later development. Through serial assessment, the clinician may observe that an infant or toddler displays one of three patterns of growth: the measured discrepancy between the child's chronological age and developmental functioning remains the same over time (normal-abnormal development), increases over time (abnormal-abnormal development), or decreases over time (catch-up growth). When catch-up growth is observed, it is considered a favorable sign for optimistic projections concerning later development.

In traditional practice, professionals have assessed the child, analyzed the information, and presented selected results to parents or caregivers, usually at a later meeting. Family-centered practice calls for a shift in this format in which parents receive information as soon as it is gathered and participate with professionals in interpreting the information (Turnbull, 1991). Turnbull gives the following suggestions for discussing information with parents:

- Discuss information with families as quickly as possible after children's special needs are suspected or formally identified.
- Use the primary language and communication style of the family, and ensure that terminology is clear and understandable.
- Set aside sufficient time for families and professionals to present information, ask questions, and provide emotional support.

- Provide families with an opportunity to decide on the appropriate family members and professionals to include in assessment conferences. Scheduling should allow for the participation of these designated team members.
- Honor family preferences for the amount of information they can absorb in one meeting. Continuing family and professional assessment feedback sessions are necessary, rather than only one or two sessions.
- Provide complete, unbiased information to families about their children's strengths and needs. Throughout the discussion of all information, families need and look for hope and encouragement. (p. 45)

These suggestions provide guidelines for including family members in the interpretation process.

CONCLUSION

This chapter has covered many topics related to child language assessment. Some assessment tools designed to evaluate infant and toddler communication have also been presented. The next chapter addresses the planning of intervention from this and other information.

Appendix 7-A

Form for Evaluating Measures of Early Communication

I. Identifying Information
   Title: _____
   Author(s): _____
   Publication date: _____
   Intended age range: _____
   Approach to assessment: ___Standardized, norm-referenced
                            ___Nonstandardized, no normative information
                            ___Criterion-referenced
                            ___Developmental scale
                            ___Other: _____
   Intended function: ___Screening of _____
                       ___Assessment of _____

II. Standardization
   A. Conditions prescribed for test administration
      1. Test situation: _____
         ___ Parent present   ___ not present
      2. Usual length of time for testing: _____
      3. Examiner training required: _____
      4. Other: _____
   B. Rules for scoring
      1. Summary of scoring procedure: _____
         _____
         _____
      2. Evaluation of scoring procedure: ___clearly explained
                                           ___unclear or ___absent
      3. Form of the score: ___percentage
                             ___age score
                             ___percentile
                             ___standard score
                             ___other: _____

C. Normative information
   1. Size of standardization sample: _____
   2. Racial/ethnic makeup: _____
   3. Proportion of male/female subjects: _____
   4. Geographic location: _____
   5. Age distribution: _____
   6. Other factors: ___urban   ___rural
                        ___handicapped   ___nonhandicapped
   7. Evaluation of the standardization sample:
      ___Adequate (representative)
      ___Inadequate (nonrepresentative)
      ___Comparable to local population
      ___Not comparable to local population
D. Procedures for systematic sampling of behavior
   1. General rules for item presentation: _____
      _____
      Evaluation: ___clear   ___unclear
   2. Order of item presentation
      ___flexible   ___inflexible
   3. Methods of sampling behavior employed:
      ___caregiver report
      ___analysis of spontaneous behavior
      ___behavioral compliance with commands
      ___question answering
      ___identification or recognition
      ___acting out or reconstruction
      ___judgment
      ___elicited imitation
      ___delayed imitation
      ___carrier phrase
      ___paraphrase
      ___other: _____
III. Materials to be used as stimuli
   ___provided   ___not provided
                  ___easy to obtain
                  ___difficult to obtain
   Evaluation:
   ___well organized in test kit   ___poorly organized
   ___familiar to most children   ___unfamiliar
   ___attractive   ___unattractive
   ___appropriate sizes   ___too large or small
   ___durable   ___easily broken
   Other comments: _____

IV. Item information

Total number of items:___

Average number of items at each age level:___

A. Processes of communication considered

___Comprehension

___Production: ___typical   ___optimal

B. Content areas assessed

___Response to auditory stimuli

___Nonverbal communication behaviors

___Evidence of oral motor abilities

___Parent-child interaction

___Play behaviors

___Understanding and use of words

___Conceptual information

___Phonological development

___Cognitive abilities

___Early word combinations (semantic relations)

___Syntax (grammatical morphemes, sentence co-ordination, etc.)

___Verbal response to questions

___Pragmatics (language functions, discourse skills, etc.)

___Auditory memory

___Other: _____

Evaluation: ___content areas are well sampled   ___not adequate

V. Information presented on reliability

Temporal (test-retest): _____

_____

Internal consistency: _____

_____

Alternate form: _____

_____

Other: _____

No information: _____

Evaluation: ___appears adequate   ___appears inadequate

VI. Information presented on validity

Content: _____

_____

Predictive: _____

_____

Concurrent: _____

_____

Construct: _____

_____

VII. Summary (overall impression of test)

_____

_____

_____

_____

_____

_____

_____

Appendix 7-B

Organizing Assessment Information Form

Content Area	Information from		Comparison to Expected Behaviors
	Formal measure(s)	**Informal measure(s)**	
Prerequisite Abilities and Conditions Oral Structure Oral Motor/Breathing			
Response to Auditory Stimuli			
Gross and Fine Motor Abilities			
Cognitive Abilities 1. Attending 2. Imitation			

Content Area	Information from		Comparison to Expected Behaviors
	Formal measure(s)	Informal measure(s)	
3. Object Constancy			
4. Symbolic Ability			
Level of Psychosocial Development			
1. Relationship with Caregiver and Others			
2. Evidence of Attachment			
3. Stranger Anxiety			
4. Separation Anxiety			
Environmental Support for Language Learning and Use			
1. "Home" Environment			
2. Experience/Stimuli			
3. Daily Activities			

Content Area	Information from		Comparison to Expected Behaviors
	Formal measure(s)	Informal measure(s)	
4. Speech-Language Models			
5. Communication Needs, Demands, Support			
6. Parent Language/Speech to the Child: Quantitative Measures (MLU, Speech Rate, Percentage of Questions, etc.)			
Communication Abilities and Use Nonverbal Communication Behaviors			
1. Eye Contact			
2. Touch			
3. Gestures			
4. Facial Gestures (Smile, Frown)			
5. Vocal Inflection			

Content Area	Information from		Comparison to Expected Behaviors
	Formal measure(s)	Informal measure(s)	
6. Phonological Development			
Receptive Language			
1. Response to Affective Communication			
2. Response to Words with Gestures			
3. Response to Words without Gestures			
4. Response to Word Combinations and Grammatical Morphemes			
5. Response to Two-Part Instructions			
6. Response to Three-Part Instructions			

Content Area	Information from		Comparison to Expected Behaviors
	Formal measure(s)	**Informal measure(s)**	
7. Understanding of Basic Concepts			
Expressive Language 1. Use of Words and Vocabulary Size			
2. Type-Token Ratio			
3. Word Combinations; Semantic/Syntactic Relationships			
4. Language Functions			

Content Area	Information from		Comparison to Expected Behaviors
	Formal measure(s)	Informal measure(s)	
5. MLU			
6. Sentence Structure			
7. Grammatical Morphemes (First 14)			
8. Expression of Basic Concepts			

Content Area	Information from		Comparison to Expected Behaviors
	Formal measure(s)	Informal measure(s)	
Ability To Answer Questions			
1. Yes/No			
2. Wh			
Fluency, Vocal Quality, Prosody			
Child's Functional Use of Vocal/Verbal Behaviors			
1. Initiation of Communication			
2. Number of Turns/Interchanges			
3. Requests for Action, Information, Goods			
4. Labeling			

Content Area	Information from		Comparison to Expected Behaviors
	Formal measure(s)	Informal measure(s)	
5. Protesting			
6. Answering			

Summary Statement

Appendix 7-C

Todd: Assessment of Child Communication

Todd and his mother, Mrs. C, were seen for three one-hour evaluation sessions during three consecutive weeks. During the first of these sessions, a 20-minute sample of mother-child interaction was videotaped. The analysis of a portion of the interaction was presented in Appendix 6-A. During the second and third sessions, Todd's language was assessed using the Sequenced Inventory of Communication Development (SICD) and the Peabody Picture Vocabulary Test (PPVT). A hearing screening was completed and a language sample was collected, as well. Todd was also observed in interaction with two other toddlers and in further interaction with his mother. Information from the evaluation sessions is summarized in Exhibit 7-C-1 using the format suggested in Chapter 7. Briefly, the formal and informal measures administered during the evaluation sessions indicated that Todd's receptive language was near age level while his expressive language was at least one year below age level. Only 40 percent of his utterances were intelligible, and more than one-third of his syllables (37.9 percent) were repeated. He passed the hearing screening. Motor abilities appeared to be adequate, although some gross motor behaviors were not well coordinated.

Appendix 9-B contains information on treatment planning and the treatment program for Todd and his family.

Exhibit 7-C-1 Organizing Assessment Information Form: Todd C.

Content Area	Information from		Comparison to Expected Behaviors
	Formal measure(s)	Informal measure(s)	
Prerequisite Abilities and Conditions			
Oral Structure		Chews crackers w/ lip closure	Structure intact
Oral Motor/Breathing		Drinks from cup unaided w/o spilling Blows bubbles	Function appears normal
Response to Auditory Stimuli	Passed P-T screening R+L Tympanometry - normal		Within Normal Limits (WNL)
Gross and Fine Motor Abilities		Walks w/some stumbling (infrequent) W-sits Rides trike (Mo's report) Manipulates small objects Builds tower w/ blocks	Probably WNL
Cognitive Abilities 1. Attending	Attends for testing- up to 30 minutes.		
2. Imitation		Spontaneous + elicited verbal + nonverbal imitation	WNL

Content Area	Information from		Comparison to
	Formal measure(s)	Informal measure(s)	Expected Behaviors
3. Object Constancy		Requests cars when out of sight	WNL
4. Symbolic Ability	Uses words	Symbolic play reported	
Level of Psychosocial Development			
1. Relationship with Caregiver and Others		Doesn't play w/new children Relates warmly to mother	Appears to be in rapproachment phase of Sep. - Ind.
2. Evidence of Attachment		Attachment behaviors to mother	
3. Stranger Anxiety		In new situation w/new child very quiet, doesn't eat snack until mo. sits w/him	
4. Separation Anxiety			
Environmental Support for Language Learning and Use			
1. "Home" Environment		Lives in single family home w/mo., fa. & 5 y-o sister	
2. Experience/Stimuli		Mo. provides learning-oriented toys, outings, etc.	
3. Daily Activities		Spends day w/mo., 3 days/wk another 2 y.o. is in the home. Plays w/5 y.o. sister in PM	

Content Area	Information from		Comparison to Expected Behaviors
	Formal measure(s)	Informal measure(s)	
4. Speech-Language Models		Parents, Sister, Grandparents	
5. Communication Needs, Demands, Support		Mo. interprets unintelligible ut.	
6. Parent Language/Speech to the Child: Quantitative Measures (MLU, Speech Rate, Percentage of Questions, etc.)		Mo's: MLU=5.42 M. SPM=350 % Sem, R.=40.9% % Acc=47.7%	3-4 M. would be more helpful; Decrease to 230 or lower; Increase; Increase
Communication Abilities and Use Nonverbal Communication Behaviors			
1. Eye Contact		Often used to indicate desired object	WNL
2. Touch		Little touching	
3. Gestures		Few	
4. Facial Gestures (Smile, Frown)		Normal use	
5. Vocal Inflection		Normal use	

Content Area	Information from		Comparison to Expected Behaviors
	Formal measure(s)	Informal measure(s)	
6. Phonological Development		Phonemes produced in Lang Sample: Initial: /j, n, w, g, m, k, h, t, b/ Final: /m, r, k/ 40% of syllables intelligible	
Receptive Language			
1. Response to Affective Communication	SICD Score; RCA = 32 MO at CA = 33 Mo.	Responds to Mo's tone of voice	WNL
2. Response to Words with Gestures	Passed Items on SICD		
3. Response to Words without Gestures	2 out of 3 passed on SICD PPVT Score 2 Mo. above age		
4. Response to Word Combinations and Grammatical Morphemes	Follows 1-Part commands (SICD) " commands for prep. in, on, under (not beside) Questionable (unreliable) response to plural		
5. Response to Two-Part Instructions	Follows 2-Part commands (40 Mo. Lev.)		
6. Response to Three-Part Instructions	Not tested		

Content Area	Information from		Comparison to Expected Behaviors
	Formal measure(s)	Informal measure(s)	
7. Understanding of Basic Concepts	Body parts ✓ / In, on, under ✓ / Fails: Colors, Numbers, Big & Little		
Expressive Language 1. Use of Words and Vocabulary Size	SICD Score; ECA=20 Mo.	MLU = 1.40 Mor. / 33 words heard / Mo. reports 50	About 1 yr below age level / Below Age Level (BAL)
2. Type-Token Ratio		.35	.50 Normal
3. Word Combinations; Semantic/Syntactic Relationships		Few combinations / Range of Sem. Rel. expressed in 1-WD ut. / -Most agreement ("yeah") & attribution	
4. Language Functions		Most responses to questions & requests / Also labels / Few requests	

Content Area	Information from		Comparison to
	Formal measure(s)	Informal measure(s)	Expected Behaviors
5. MLU		1.40 M.	
6. Sentence Structure		2 WD ut. Infrequent	
7. Grammatical Morphemes (First 14)		None apparent	
8. Expression of Basic Concepts			Same color names (often incorrect)

Content Area	Information from		Comparison to Expected Behaviors
	Formal measure(s)	Informal measure(s)	
Ability To Answer Questions			
1. Yes/No	Correct resp. on SIDc	Answers readily w/ yeah & no	
2. Wh	Answers on "what" Q.		
Fluency, Vocal Quality, Prosody		37.9% of syllables Repeated - High Rep. rate Voice WNL	
Child's Functional Use of Vocal/Verbal Behaviors			
1. Initiation of Communication		Seldom	
2. Number of Turns/Interchanges		Not measured	
3. Requests for Action, Information, Goods		Seldom	
4. Labeling		Some	

Content Area	Information from		Comparison to Expected Behaviors
	Formal measure(s)	Informal measure(s)	
5. Protesting		By saying no	
6. Answering		Frequent	

Summary Statement

Age appropriate receptive language
Expressive language about 1-yr below age level
- Poor intelligibility
- Marked repetitions
Phonological DEV. - Age appropriate - ?
Prerequisite abilities appear intact
Parent language model & responses: fast rate, long MLU, non-accepting

8

Planning Intervention with and for the Family

Previous sections of this book have discussed the idea of family members as equal partners in the intervention process and their potential empowerment from this involvement. The family's participation in assessment of the infant's/ toddler's communication has been demonstrated to be crucial to the professional's collection of accurate and complete information on the child's abilities and the context in which those abilities were acquired and will develop. While family members' participation is important to all phases of assessment and treatment, it may be that it is most important in the planning of intervention. Treatment can only be family centered if the family's values and priorities are considered. If the clinician is to act as a successful consultant to the family, family members must participate in the early phases of the consultation—assessment and planning.

The process of formally planning intervention is an important one for both professionals and family members. The team not only decides what the next appropriate area(s) and levels of development are and how best to help the child get there, the team members also educate one another. That is, they continue to share information concerning the specific child and their understanding of development in general. This information may have been partially tapped in the assessment process, but with the practical, real-life focus of planning, much more information may surface.

It is also in the planning process that team members' expectations become clear. As they consider goals, objectives, and expected outcomes, important exchanges about what seems to be possible for this child, right now, may take place.

Family members' cooperation and participation in treatment may be won or lost during this planning stage. If their perceived needs, values, and priorities for their child are appreciated by other team members and if they are respected as equals, they may be able to contribute in many positive ways.

FAMILY INVOLVEMENT IN PLANNING

It would certainly be a mistake to assume that all parents or other family members want to be integrally involved in each high-risk or impaired infant's treatment on a day-to-day basis. It is probably true, however, that families usually want to be involved on the level at which they perceive themselves capable (in terms of time, temperament, and skills) of being involved.

The small body of research into parent preferences for involvement in treatment supports the notion that clinicians should not assume a desire for complete involvement in all aspects of intervention on the part of all families. Andrews, Andrews, and Shearer (1989), in a survey of 1,684 families with children receiving speech-language services in the schools, found that respondents varied in their desire for involvement in treatment. Fifty-one percent of the respondents were interested in a family approach to treatment in which parents would give input and learn treatment techniques for use at home. The typical respondent in this group ". . . tended not to have a full understanding of the nature of the problem and believed that the problem had not improved significantly . . . [and] was rather severe" (p. 394). These parents were often single, and the children tended to be young, have few siblings, and have language disorder as their predominant problem.

Further, Turnbull and Turnbull (1986) reviewed literature on the topic of parent preference for involvement in treatment and found that, in general, parents prefer to have informal contacts with program personnel. Parents in the studies reviewed preferred frequent contacts and liked to give and receive information more than they liked to be in an active decision-making role.

There are a number of family system-related issues that may affect family involvement in planning for intervention and in intervention itself. It is important to note that system characteristics can apply to families from any culture. In fact, consideration of the way families operate as systems is one way to view cultural similarities and differences. In considering these system-related issues, it may be helpful to review the idea of the family as a system with its components in dynamic balance with one another. As noted earlier, any system, and especially the family system, tends to resist change because it throws the system into a state of disequilibrium. Planning of intervention is, of course, planning for change, therefore the family system may resist this process as an unconscious defense against this disequilibrium. As Lund (1986) states,

> . . . it is not that [family members] wish to keep the child "impaired" but rather that changing behavior toward that family member brings with it changes in the whole family system. Having the identified child as the focus of family concern may in some cases keep the rest of the system operating smoothly; changes in the child may throw off the balance and cause stress to be manifested elsewhere. (p. 425)

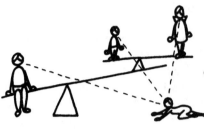

Every family system operates according to certain rules that serve to maintain its balance. In addition, each family is characterized by the degree of cohesion and adaptability of its members' relationships and interactions (Turnbull & Turnbull, 1986) (see Chapter 1). A family's degree of cohesion, the emotional bonding and degree of interdependence of its members, has been conceptualized as being on a continuum from "enmeshment" to "disengagement" (Minuchin, 1974). In an enmeshed family there is little differentiation between family members and their roles. There is a high degree of interdependence. The opposite is true of disengaged families. Their members function independently and have highly differentiated roles. Probably the best functioning families exist at a midpoint on this continuum with family members experiencing both close relationship and a sense of autonomy (Turnbull & Turnbull, 1986).

Understanding family cohesion helps us to recognize some of the issues that are important to the family's involvement in treatment planning. Cohesion relates to the family's "boundary rules" (Lund, 1986). These rules dictate who can participate in an activity and how the participants relate to each other and to those not involved in the activity. They also dictate what activities family members should do on their own and what functions they will share with or assign to outside forces. Understanding these boundary rules may help us to understand why one family has difficulty letting outsiders help them to plan for ways to facilitate language development (teaching a child to talk is seen exclusively as a family function) and another family can happily collaborate for treatment planning (language-learning difficulties are seen as problems that need outside or "expert" input). An enmeshed family may have particular difficulty letting outsiders participate with a family member, while a disengaged family may be all too willing to turn over the treatment to a professional (Lund, 1986).

Another issue to be considered in terms of family cohesion is the effect of the interventions we plan for certain families. Some interventions, such as intensive parental involvement in treatment activities, may encourage enmeshment with the child. It is important for us to be aware of the effects that this may have on the family system (Turnbull & Turnbull, 1986). Especially in family systems that tend to be disengaged, the expectation of a high level of involvement with one member may create stress in the family system. Frequently, suggestions that require a greater degree of interaction than the family can comfortably manage will be ignored or "forgotten."

The degree of adaptability of the family system relates to the family's ability to change in response to external and internal stresses (Turnbull & Turnbull,

1986) (see Chapter 1). Like family cohesion, adaptability can be viewed as a continuum; rigid families are at one extreme, and chaotic families are at the other. Rigid families are very controlled and structured, allowing little change to take place. Chaotic families are much less structured, often having few rules and those that they do have either change frequently or are not enforced. As with cohesion, the most functional families exist at a midpoint on the adaptability continuum, neither too rigid nor too chaotic.

Because the family's ability to adapt to change is important in the intervention process, it is an issue which professionals must take into consideration. It is important to identify the person(s) in the family who control family responses to pressures for change and to involve them in planning for intervention. Treatment plans must also consider the family's capacity for adapting to the changes that are required. A rigid family may demand much more gradual objectives to reach treatment goals than a more adaptable family would (Turnbull & Turnbull, 1986).

Two other family system-related issues that may require some consideration are alignment and equitability (Lund, 1986). In healthy families, alliances between family members are formed and dissolved frequently in response to various situations. In some less functional families, these alliances may be more stable or may serve to designate one family member as the source of "the problem." Alignment may also be an issue when a clinician forms an alliance with a family member (Lund, 1986).

Equitability also plays a role in treatment planning and execution within the family system. Families have rules about what's fair treatment and "who owes what to whom" (Lund, 1986, p. 425). The family that must plan for a child with an impairment may have many issues that require special attention to the maintenance of equitable treatment for all members.

All of these issues may play a role at one time or another in treatment planning and especially in the family's desire and ability to participate in this process. A great deal of sensitivity and awareness on the part of the clinician may be required to help family members to participate fully in the planning process.

While family participation in planning for intervention may help to ensure the success of treatment efforts, that is not the only reason for facilitating this participation. Under P.L. 99-457, family members must be included on the service planning team. The law specifies that after a multidisciplinary assessment of the infant's or toddler's needs, a written IFSP must be developed in a reasonable period of time by a multidisciplinary team which includes the parent or guardian of the child. The content of this IFSP was discussed in Chapter 4.

Bailey and Wolery (1989) point out that parents have the right not only to participate in assessment and treatment planning, but also to truly understand what the results of the assessment mean. In addition, Bailey and Wolery (1989) noted that parents are often unaware of their rights regarding assessment and planning. When this is the case, it is the clinician's responsibility to teach parents about their rights. With some families, the services of an interpreter may be required to ensure that the family understands and participates in the planning process. Further, the provisions of P.L. 99-457 should be met at the level of the intent of the law, not just the letter of the law. This will often include making sure that parents understand not only their legal rights, but also the options that are available to them and their child to meet those rights (Bailey & Wolery, 1989).

Perhaps the most important issue related to family involvement in treatment planning is the benefits that acrue to both the child and the family. As noted earlier, change throws the family system into disequilibrium. Because of this, families tend to resist even beneficial change. This is especially true when that change is imposed from outside the system. When family members can be involved in planning the interventions that are to institute change they are more likely to be able to collaborate in that intervention. This may be because they feel more capable and in control of the situation (empowered), or because they fully understand the reasons for the intervention. Whatever the reasons, family involvement seems to benefit the treatment process.

Mori (1983) cites several purposes that are served by involving families in the intervention for a child.

> The family-child relationship can be greatly improved. Intervention is far more effective when families understand and meet the child's and their own needs. Parents benefit from the exchange of information with professionals and others who have had similar experiences. Finally, the program itself may benefit because families may become advocates in the community for stronger programs. (pp. 214–215)

Given all of these considerations and benefits, clinicians need ways to facilitate family involvement in treatment planning. Once the clinician knows the family well enough to recognize its members' roles, boundaries, rules, and characteristics of cohesion, he or she can begin to draw family members into the planning process at a level that is appropriate to each member and to the family system.

Not all families wish to or are capable of being integrally involved in all phases of their infant's or toddler's assessment and intervention. The desire for involvement may be different from culture to culture. For example, while Asian Americans tend to be very concerned about their children's schooling, they may expect respected professionals to take control of the treatment or educational situation rather than seeking their input (Cheng, 1987). Additionally, some families are coping at the limit of their abilities just managing day-to-day chores. They may find it difficult to take on any additional tasks or even the responsibility of making decisions. Therefore, "optimal" involvement may differ greatly from family to family. For some families, contributing information, staying informed about treatment progress, and getting the child to treatment sessions may be the most manageable level of involvement. Others may wish to be involved in all aspects of assessment, planning, and intervention. The right level of involvement is whatever level best supports and promotes family functioning to help the infant or toddler develop. Family involvement is discussed further in Chapter 9.

It may be helpful at the outset of the treatment planning process to clarify family members' perceptions of what treatment is all about—what the general objectives and possible outcomes may be as well as the kinds of intervention that might be appropriate. With some families, it may be appropriate to have an open discussion of how intrusive or intensive the treatment program will be. It is helpful to put the families in touch with other families who are already involved in the treatment process.

Bailey (1987) and Bailey and Wolery (1989) have discussed some basic practices that clinicians can use to facilitate "collaborative goal-setting." Bailey and Wolery (1989) state,

> These include (a) viewing the family as a functioning system within a society of systems, (b) assessing family needs and attempting to establish goals and interventions that accommodate those needs . . . , (c) employing effective interviewing and listening skills throughout the assessment and while planning intervention, (d) negotiating goals and interventions because of potentially different values, and (e) filling the case-management role for families by helping them secure the services they need. (p. 493)

The clinician's role in facilitation may also entail providing parents with information that helps them to participate knowledgeably in meetings, and actively seeking family input that contributes to decision making (Bailey & Wolery, 1989). Clear and open communication is probably the most important tool that the professional can use in facilitating family involvement.

Mori (1983) has also stressed the value of clinicians focusing on the ". . . needs of the parents as individuals and members of a family unit" (p. 210). Mori further states,

> If the training of parents to assume new or more involved roles as teachers of their children is to be successful, it must assist them in meeting their basic needs as individuals, as well as their needs as parents. Parents whose own basic needs are met will certainly be in a better position to meet the new needs or challenges that arise in being

the parent of a handicapped child. Thus . . . the trainers of parents must first recognize them as adult members of a dynamic ecological construct. Furthermore, these professionals must be aware of parents' needs for self-esteem and self-actualization. (p. 211)

DESIRED OUTCOMES: TARGETS FOR TREATMENT

Public Law 99-457 (1986) specifies that the IFSP contain "a statement of the major outcomes expected to be achieved for the infant and toddler and the family, and the criteria, procedures, and timelines used to determine the degree to which progress toward achieving the outcomes are being made and whether modifications or revisions of the outcomes or services are necessary" (p. 2.10). These "outcomes" are often stated in terms of long-term goals and short-term objectives as most of us have written them since P.L. 94-142 helped us to improve our accountability with their use. However, Kramer, McGonigel, and Kaufmann (1991) stress the importance of differentiating between IFSP outcomes and IEP goals and objectives. According to Kramer et al., an outcome is "a statement of the changes family members want to see for their child or themselves . . . [and is] functionally stated in terms of what is to occur (process) and what is expected as a result of these actions (product)" (p. 57). These outcomes are written in the language that the family uses to talk about these desired changes.

Treatment goals usually state an expected outcome that can be achieved over an extended period of time, while treatment objectives provide short-term targets that move the child closer to the behavior specified in the goal. Objectives are written in a format that allows the clinician to readily evaluate whether or not they have been achieved. Each objective tells what (the desired behavioral outcome) will be done by whom (the target individual or group) under what conditions and to what extent (the criteria for evaluating the behavior's reliability, e.g., percentage of time correct, number of times a behavior is exhibited in a certain timeframe, and the date by which it is to be measured). This behaviorally based language is very helpful clinically, but it may not be meaningful to families.

For example, the Reynolds family was finding it very upsetting for 19-month-old Mona to cry and point when she wanted things. They often could not figure out what she wanted and everyone was feeling frustrated. The outcome would be stated as: the Reynolds want some help teaching Mona to use words so that she will ask for the food and toys that she wants. If this were stated as a behavioral objective it might read: Mr. and Mrs. Reynolds will model single-word utterances for Mona 90 percent of the time when she nonverbally indicates a desired object during a sample of interaction recorded on January 15, 1992.

The behavioral objective gives important information, but the professional jargon may make it seem foreign to the family. Kramer et al. (1991) note that some programs are opting to write both family-generated outcomes and behavioral objectives. This combination may well provide the best means of meeting both family and professional needs.

Bailey and Simeonsson (1988) cite four reasons for specifying goals and objectives for treatment:

1. to meet the legal requirements of P.L. 99-457
2. to enhance the effectiveness of intervention by providing a focus for intervention efforts
3. to provide a means of monitoring progress
4. to communicate expectations.

The goals and objectives written for infants and toddlers in accordance with P.L. 99-457 differ in another respect from the goals and objectives written for older children under P.L. 94-142. While the child is still the primary target for the intervention efforts, P.L. 99-457 requires a statement of family strengths and needs as they relate to the child's development, and of the outcomes expected for both the child and the family (Bailey & Simeonsson, 1988). Thus, the child is no longer the only target for treatment; the family is to be considered when goals are written.

DEVELOPING INDIVIDUALIZED FAMILY-CENTERED GOALS

The framework of the IFSP provides a well-structured process for developing family-centered goals. Campbell (1990, May) emphasizes that it is the process of developing family-centered goals that is important, rather than the document that results. The IFSP document that is generated is only the written record of the process. She states, "The process that results in the completion of the written IFSP document is one where professionals enhance a family's ability to become active planners for their children" (p. 7).

According to the final regulations for P.L. 99-457 as set forth in the *Federal Register,* June 22, 1989, the individualized family service plan must: (1) be developed jointly by the family and qualified personnel, (2) be based on multidisciplinary evaluation and assessment of the child and family (family assessment is voluntary on the part of the family), and (3) "include services necessary to enhance the development of the child and the capacity of the family to meet the special needs of the child" (p. 26320).

The IFSP must be reviewed every six months, or more frequently if necessary or requested by the family, to evaluate the progress being made toward the desired outcomes. An annual meeting must be conducted to evaluate the IFSP and to revise its provisions if necessary.

All IFSP meetings must be scheduled at times and in places that are convenient for the family, and are to be conducted in the family's native language or normal mode of communication (e.g., sign language). These meetings must include the parent(s) of the child, any other family members requested by the parent(s), a nonfamily-member advocate if requested by the family, the service coordinator (also called case manager in some programs), person(s) who conducted the evaluations and assessments of the child and family, and persons who will provide services to the child or family.

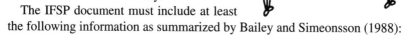

The IFSP document must include at least the following information as summarized by Bailey and Simeonsson (1988):

1. A statement of the infant's or toddler's present levels of physical development, cognitive development, language and speech development, psychosocial development, and self-help skills, based on acceptable objective criteria. . . .

2. A statement of the family's strengths and needs related to enhancing the development of the family's handicapped infant or toddler. . . .

3. A statement of major goals for the infant or toddler and the family, and the criteria, procedures, and timelines used to measure progress toward these goals and determine if modifications of goals or services are necessary. . . .

4. A statement of specific early intervention services necessary to meet the unique needs of the infant or toddler and the family, including the frequency, intensity [meaning the number of days or sessions that will be provided, the length of each session, and whether sessions are group or individual sessions], and method of delivering services. . . .

5. The projected dates for initiation of services and the anticipated duration of such services. . . .

6. The name of the case manager from the profession most immediately relevant to the infant's or toddler's and the family's needs, who will be responsible for implementing the plan and coordinating with other agencies and persons. . . .

7. The steps to be taken supporting the transition of the handicapped toddler to services provided for preschoolers to the extent such services are considered appropriate. (pp. 245-247)

States that have developed formats for IFSP documents have produced different forms to cover these components. Two examples of these forms, one adopted for Arkansas and one for Maryland, are included in Appendix 8-A. These formats are presented only as illustrations of different forms and not with any intent to evaluate their content or structure.

The following eight-step process for IFSP development is based on the work of Campbell (1990, May) and McGonigel, Kaufman, and Hurth (1991):

Step 1: Statement of Philosophy and Values. Staff members of each early intervention program establish and record a program philosophy concerning families, child-rearing practices, etc., and make this statement available to families who may use their services (Campbell, 1990, May).

Step 2: First Contacts with the Family. Professionals meet with the child and family to establish rapport, gather and provide information, and screen the child to determine the need for further evaluation (Campbell, 1990, May). McGonigel et al. (1991) stress that this may be the most important time for the parent-professional relationship. It is the time when professionals learn the family's idea of how early intervention will be involved in its life and what family priorities are concerning this child and other family members. It is also the time to identify who constitutes the family.

If the child does not need services at this time, referrals or plans to rescreen the child at a later date may be made. If the child is found to need services but the family decides not to participate in the program at this time, arrangements may be made to recontact the family in the future and professionals may review the first contacts to ascertain whether parents received appropriate information and support (McGonigel et al., 1991).

Step 3: Assessment Planning. The family and staff plan the assessment of the child. At this time, the professional team gathers information concerning child characteristics (health, development, etc.), family preferences for involvement, and any special kinds of information that family members would like to learn from the assessment. Family input helps to determine the participants, measures, and procedures used in the evaluation (McGonigel et al., 1991).

Step 4: Child Assessment/Evaluation. One or more professionals evaluate the child in the five areas listed in the description of IFSP content above. This evaluation determines the child's eligibility for services and provides a positive description of abilities in each of the developmental areas. Ongoing child and family assessments are then done to determine services needed (Campbell, 1990, May). Family members are included in all discussions of the child's evaluation; professionals use terms that family members understand and prefer and avoid jargon (McGonigel et al., 1991).

Step 5: Determining Desired Outcomes. Professionals and family members collaborate to determine desired treatment outcomes for the child and family. Family priorities are of prime importance in this process. The written document that results from this step includes information about the child's current developmental abilities, the desired outcomes, and early intervention services that will be provided (Campbell, 1990, May).

Step 6: Ongoing Child and Family Assessment. Desired outcomes are analyzed to determine treatment objectives and strategies to attain the outcomes. Interested families are helped to identify their strengths and needs using interview procedures that may be supplemented by formal or informal family needs assessment tools (Campbell, 1990, May; McGonigel et al., 1991).

Step 7: Implementation. The plan outlined by the IFSP is put into effect with service providers developing detailed plans for activities and strategies to work toward the objectives related to each desired outcome. The family and staff carry out the activities and strategies. The services are coordinated (Campbell, 1990; McGonigel et al., 1991).

Step 8: Review and Update of the IFSP Document. Family members and the service coordinator evaluate program outcomes. The IFSP is reviewed and updated at least every six months. A meeting to revise the document is held annually (Campbell, 1990, May; McGonigel et al., 1991).

These steps provide a general guide to the IFSP process. They cover all areas except the transition plan required by P.L. 99-457. This transition plan is only necessary in the year prior to the child's third birthday, when the child would become eligible for preschool services under Part B of P.L. 94-142, or in the event of relocation of the family. The plan for transition would not be part of the initial IFSP process for most families.

Determining Desired Outcomes

The portion of the process covered in Step 5 above sounds deceptively simple. In fact, it is often a complicated and demanding task for professionals and family members to collaborate in the determination of outcomes that are appropriate for the child and family. There are two basic approaches to the determination of these outcomes. One approach begins with the family's hopes and expectations and works toward strategies to attain these outcomes. This has been called a "top down" approach (Campbell, 1990, May). The other method begins with assessment information and identifies strengths and weaknesses. This information is used to determine goals that relate to identified deficits, but that may have little to do with what the family really desires for the child. Campbell (1990, May) refers to this strategy as a "bottom up" approach. Both of these methods may be useful and appropriate ways to determine what goals are important for a given child and family. Both strategies will be discussed below, beginning with the determination of family priorities.

Identifying Family Priorities

This approach to determining desired outcomes begins with questions such as, "What's important to this family? What are their hopes and expectations for this child? What do they wish the child could do or have that would make family life better? What would help them to help this child?" As stated in an earlier chapter of this book, families may sometimes find it difficult to form expectations for a sick child or a child with an impairment because their original expectations were not met. When this is the case they may defer to the professionals involved with the child, or they may generate what seem to be unrealistic desires. In either case, the clinicians are faced with the difficulty of respecting the family's values and helping family members to ascertain priorities rather than simply imposing their own.

Campbell (1990, May) suggests that professionals help family members to generate outcomes by asking them to take the lead in describing their child's abilities. Professionals can then supplement the parents' descriptions with additional information on what the child is able to do. After this positive introduction, a clinician may help family members to generate desired outcomes by giving examples of outcomes from other families. Campbell provided the following suggestion:

> Professionals provide a background for families through statements such as "a mother told me yesterday that one thing she would like for her son to be able to do is to go to Sunday school at church. What types of activities is your family interested in having _____ do?" In ways such as this, professionals establish that the IFSP will be based on *family-desired outcomes* (emphasis in original) for their children, rather than a compilation of goals and objectives from professionals. (p. 14)

After family priorities have been recorded, professionals may suggest other appropriate outcomes for the family's consideration. Even when outcomes suggested by the family do not seem appropriate to the professionals, their task is to attempt to understand why the family values that outcome and why they have expressed it. It may be that the family is seeking clarification of what they really can expect as an outcome of treatment (e.g., is it realistic to hope that John will talk clearly by the time he is three years old?), or it may be that there is an underlying ability that can be achieved in some other way that is at the core of the parents' stated desire. Campbell (1990, May) presents a clear example of this issue:

> Professionals do not judge the validity or feasibility of outcomes established by families but rather attempt to understand exactly what outcome(s) a family desires. . . . When families of children with very severe disabilities request performance of skills that do not appear to be "realistic" for the child, given the degree of disability, professionals need to expand and inform families of the ways in which this outcome may be achieved. For example, if a family of a child with a severe physical disability establishes walking as an outcome, the professional reshapes this statement by saying something like "It sounds important to you for _____ to be able to get around the house without your help. Walking independently may not be easy for _____ to learn but getting around the house by himself is something we can work on by teaching him to _____ (e.g., use a walker, motorized car, tot sized wheel chair, etc.)." In this way professionals respect the content of a family's message without getting tied to the specific way in which that outcome might be obtained. (p. 15)

This kind of sensitivity to the family's values and desires requires experience and clinical prowess. It takes both skill and insight to respond in a helpful and supportive way that allows the family to develop understanding of what is feasible and a set of outcomes that satisfy their expectations. But only when the outcomes and goals fit with family values will the family fully accept and follow through on program objectives (Bailey & Simeonsson, 1988).

Generating Treatment Outcomes from Evaluation Information

The second approach to determining outcomes, which was introduced above, begins at a different point. Rather than trying to ascertain what the family wants a child to be able to do, this approach begins with the data from the evaluation of the child's strengths and needs. While this approach is more child-centered than family-centered, it is a reasonable way to determine developmentally appropriate goals and objectives. When this approach is combined with the process of identifying family-desired outcomes, it can be an important part of the establishment of a suitable focus for services.

By comparing the data from the evaluation of the child's abilities with normative data the clinician can identify areas of competence and deficit. Goals and objectives can be written to address any significant areas of deficit. We can further specify goals to eliminate any factors that limit the child's ability to communicate (e.g., positioning that makes respiration and breath support for speech difficult), or factors that produce a breakdown in communication (e.g., excessive parental demands for correct pronunciation from a child who has problems with oral motor coordination). We may also specify goals to increase factors and situations that promote better communication (e.g., parents following the child's lead in play and communication and positive responding to the child's attempts to use words). Lund (1986) referred to these goals that actively seek change as "first-order" effects of intervention.

Second-order effects of intervention include those which are indirect results of intervention (Lund, 1986). Goals related to these second-order changes seek to increase the positive and decrease the negative effects of change. For example, a second-order change which may result from a child's increased ability to make verbal requests might be an older sibling's jealousy of the child's increased attention from the parents. To decrease this effect, the sibling might be put in charge of responding to some of the child's requests with increased positive attention being paid to the sibling for being such a big help. The overriding goal here is to help the family to support the change that is occurring in the child while keeping the family system in functional balance (Lund, 1986).

CONCLUSION

However the desired outcomes are established, all goals and objectives that are generated from them should be evaluated for age and developmental appropriateness, functional and social validity, achievability, and congruence with family values and priorities (Bailey & Wolery, 1989). Those goals that are of highest priority for the family become the first targets and are the first to be scheduled for treatment. The persons and resources necessary to work toward the goals are identified in the IFSP document, along with the procedures, criteria, and timelines that will be used to evaluate the progress toward these goals.

Chapter 9 explores the implementation of family-centered goals in treatment of communication disorders.

Appendix 8-A

Examples of IFSP Forms

Arkansas Department of Human Services
Division of Developmental Disabilities Services
INDIVIDUAL FAMILY SERVICE PLAN

Family Name _____ Facilitator _____

FAMILY MEMBER	DATE OF BIRTH	AGE	RELATIONSHIP

CHILD'S FUNCTIONING LEVEL		CHILD'S STRENGTHS
AREAS		

FAMILY STRENGTHS

FAMILY/CHILD INVOLVEMENT

DDS-5201 (9/89)

Family _____

PROJECTED DATES & INITIALS	NEED (Goals)	SOURCE OF SUPPORT/RESOURCE (Method)

H	NA/Parent Initials	No Longer a Need, Goal, Aspiration, or Project		2	Unchanged; Still a Need, Goal, Aspiration, or Project
	1	Unresolved or Worse; Unattainable			

Family _____ Page Number _____

ACTION (Frequency and Intensity)	EVALUATION DATE AND H RATING INITIAL BELOW									

3	Resolved or Attained; But Not to the Family's Satisfaction	4	Unresolved or Partially Attained, But Improved
		5/Parent Initials	Resolved or Attained to the Family's Satisfaction

Peer Contact:
(hours/week)_____ Children without disabilities_____ Children with disabilities_____

Transition Plan (to be filled in 6 months prior to new placement)

Preschool Service (location) _____

Date To Begin _____

Services/Supports Required _____

_____

_____

DATE	NOTES/COMMENTS

This IFSP is reflective of our families' needs and concerns. We are in agreement with the goals and with the placement made.

_____ _____
Parent/Guardian Signature   Date

_____ _____
Team Members As per Parents Request   Date

MARYLAND INDIVIDUALIZED FAMILY SERVICE PLAN (IFSP)

Child's Name: _____   Phone: _____   Address: _____

Child's Birthdate: _____

Parent(s) Name(s): _____   Phone: _____   Address: _____

Case Manager's Name: _____   Phone: _____   Agency/Address: _____

REFERRAL DATE: _____

MEETING DATE: _____

IFSP TYPE:
_____ Interim
_____ Initial
_____ Annual Evaluation

TRANSITION PLAN ATTACHED: _____ Yes   _____ Not Applicable

PART 1: IFSP TEAM

Parent(s)/Family:

I (We) have had the opportunity to participate in the development of this IFSP. I (We) have been informed of my (our) rights under this program, through receipt of the Early Intervention System Parents' Rights Brochure. I (We) understand the plan, and parental rights, and ((we) give permission to implement this plan.

_____
Signature of Parent(s)/Guardian/Surrogate   Date

Other IFSP Meeting Participants:

Each agency or person who has a direct role in the provision of early intervention services is responsible for making a good faith effort to assist each eligible child and their family in achieving the outcomes on the child's IFSP.

_____   _____
Signature/Interim Case Manager   Agency & Title

_____   _____
Signature/Case Manager   Agency & Title

_____   _____
Signature/Lead Agency Representative   Agency & Title

_____   _____
Signature   Agency & Title

Date Form Completed: _____

MARYLAND INFANTS AND TODDLERS DATA ADD/CHANGE FORM

Child's Name: _____   Birthdate: _____

* *

CHILD AND FAMILY INFORMATION

Child's Social Security #: _____   Child's Medical Assistance #: _____
Child's Address: _____   Child's Phone #: _____
Mother's Name: _____   Mother's Birthdate: _____   Mother's Social Security #: _____
Mother's Address: _____   Mother's Phone #: _____
Father's Name: _____
Father's Address: _____   Father's Phone #: _____
Other Family/Contact Name: _____   Relationship to Child: _____
Other Family/Contact Address: _____   Other Phone #: _____

* *

CHILD STATUS

_____ Inactive: _____   Inactive as of (date): _____

_____ Deceased   _____ Out of county   _____ Other (Please specify) _____
_____ No longer eligible   _____ Parent withdrawal
_____ Transition (Part B/Other)   _____ Whereabouts unknown

* *

INDIVIDUALIZED FAMILY SERVICE PLAN (IFSP) REVIEW

Review Date: Review Type: Review Status: Case Manager:
_____   _____ Six month   _____ Continue IFSP   Name: _____
_____   _____ Parent request   _____ Modify IFSP   Agency: _____
_____   _____ Provider request _____ End IFSP   Phone #: _____
_____   _____ Parent/provider request   Signature: _____

_____ I (We) have had the opportunity to participate in the review of this IFSP and approve the review status indicated above.
_____ I (We) give permission to the early intervention program to implement attached outcome and service revisions.

_____   _____
Signature of Parent(s)/Guardian/Surrogate   Date

Child's Name: _____

PART II: CHILD'S DEVELOPMENTAL STATUS AND FAMILY INFORMATION

A. CHILD'S PRESENT LEVELS OF DEVELOPMENT

Area	Date of Procedure	Chron. Age	Age Level/ Age Range
Cognitive			
Speech/Language			
Psychosocial			
Self-Help			
Health Status:			
(Primary Health Care Provider)			
+			

Area	Date Procedure	Chron. Age	Age Level/ Age Range
Physical:			
Fine Motor			
Gross Motor			
Hearing			
+			
Vision			
+			

+ Indicates space for recording status of child's hearing, vision, and health

B. CHILD'S STRENGTHS AND NEEDS

Strengths:

Needs:

C. FAMILY STRENGTHS AND NEEDS RELATED TO ENHANCING THE CHILD'S DEVELOPMENT (voluntary on part of family)

Strengths:

Needs:

Child's Name: _____

PART III: CHILD/FAMILY OUTCOMES RELATED TO CHILD DEVELOPMENT (Related to eligible services under Part H)

Outcome #

Strategies/Activities:

Criteria/Timelines:

Person(s) Responsible:
(Name, Title, Phone #)

Ending Date:

Outcome #

Strategies/Activities:

Criteria/Timelines:

Person(s) Responsible:
(Name, Title, Phone #)

Ending Date:

Outcome #

Strategies/Activities:

Criteria/Timelines:

Person(s) Responsible:
(Name, Title, Phone #)

Ending Date:

Child's Name: _____

PART IV: EARLY INTERVENTION PROGRAM SERVICES (Eligible services under Part H)

Service: _____ Addition Date: _____
  Modification Date: _____
  Ending Date: _____

Provider Name:

Provider Agency:

Frequency: **Intensity:** **Basis:** _____ **Group** _____ **Individual**

Location: **Financial Responsibility:**

Initiation Date: **Projected Duration:**

Service: _____ Addition Date: _____
  Modification Date: _____
  Ending Date: _____

Provider Name:

Provider Agency:

Frequency: **Intensity:** **Basis:** _____ **Group** _____ **Individual**

Location: **Financial Responsibility:**

Initiation Date: **Projected Duration:**

Service: _____ Addition Date: _____
  Modification Date: _____
  Ending Date: _____

Provider Name:

Provider Agency:

Frequency: **Intensity:** **Basis:** _____ **Group** _____ **Individual**

Location: **Financial Responsibility:**

Initiation Date: **Projected Duration:**

Child's Name:

PART V: OTHER CHILD/FAMILY OUTCOMES (Related to non-required services under Part H)

Outcome #

Strategies/Activities:

Criteria/Timelines:

Person(s) Responsible:
(Name, Title, Phone #)

Ending Date:

Outcome #

Strategies/Activities:

Criteria/Timelines:

Person(s) Responsible:
(Name, Title, Phone #)

Ending Date:

Outcome #

Strategies/Activities:

Criteria/Timelines:

Person(s) Responsible:
(Name, Title, Phone #)

Ending Date:

Child's Name: _____

PART VI: SERVICE LINKAGES FOR OTHER CHILD/FAMILY OUTCOMES (Nonrequired services under Part H)

Service: _____

Primary Client: _____

Provider Agency: _____

Funding Source(s): _____

Addition Date: _____
Modification Date: _____
Ending Date: _____

Service: _____

Primary Client: _____

Provider Agency: _____

Funding Source(s): _____

Addition Date: _____
Modification Date: _____
Ending Date: _____

Service: _____

Primary Client: _____

Provider Agency: _____

Funding Source(s): _____

Addition Date: _____
Modification Date: _____
Ending Date: _____

Service: _____

Primary Client: _____

Provider Agency: _____

Funding Source(s): _____

Addition Date: _____
Modification Date: _____
Ending Date: _____

Service: _____

Primary Client: _____

Provider Agency: _____

Funding Source(s): _____

Addition Date: _____
Modification Date: _____
Ending Date: _____

Service: _____

Primary Client: _____

Provider Agency: _____

Funding Source(s): _____

Addition Date: _____
Modification Date: _____
Ending Date: _____

Service: _____

Primary Client: _____

Provider Agency: _____

Funding Source(s): _____

Addition Date: _____
Modification Date: _____
Ending Date: _____

Child's Name: _____

PART VII: TRANSITION PLAN

	Date Initiated	Date Completed

Transition Plan Provisions

Discuss community program options for child

Discuss community program options for family

Provide parental rights and responsibilities (i.e., procedural safeguards)

Identify, schedule, and conduct evaluations/assessments/procedures to determine eligibility for programs

Identify program options for child based on results of evaluations/assessments/procedures

Identify and implement steps to assist families in evaluating available and eligible programs and services

Identify and implement steps to assist families in accessing available and eligible programs and services

Transmit specified information to local education agency, with written consent from parents (when child will receive special education and related services - Part B)

Transmit specified information to other community programs, upon parent request

Identify and implement steps to help child adjust to and function in new environments

TRANSITION TO:

_____ Part B Services

Child Care/Enrichment

_____ In-Home Child Care
_____ School-Age Child Care
_____ Preschool Program
_____ Head Start
_____ Camps, Day/Residential
_____ Tutoring

Medical/Health

_____ Diagnostic/Advisory Clinics
_____ Equipment/Devices
_____ Home Health Care
_____ Hospitalization
_____ Immunizations
_____ Mental Health Services
_____ Primary Health Care
_____ Surgical Procedure
_____ WIC Program

Other

_____ Parent Education
_____ Support Group
_____ Recreation Program
_____ Other (specify)

9

Family-Centered Treatment

Therapeutic involvement with infants and toddlers and their families has changed over the years. Indeed, our perception of the abilities and needs of very young children have changed remarkably. As recently as the first half of the twentieth century infants were thought to be generally passive and incompetent beings. They were assumed to be blind and deaf at birth, asocial and unresponsive for several months, and psychologically neutral, having no particular needs in that realm. Parents were seen as providers of basic, physical care and, most importantly, discipline (Trout, 1987). Interactions with infants were to be calm and not overly stimulating events, as illustrated by this quote from Emmet Holt, MD, from the 1898 edition of his text for physicians, *Diseases of Infancy & Childhood,*

> Playing with young children, stimulating to laughter and exciting them by sights, sounds or movements until they shriek with apparent delight, may be a source of amusement to fond parents and admiring spectators, but it is almost invariably an injury to the child. It is the plain duty of the physician to enlighten parents upon this point and insist that the infant shall be kept quiet, and that all such playing and romping as has been referred to shall, during the first year at least, be absolutely prohibited. (cited in Trout, 1987, p. 15)

Fortunately, research findings have helped us to become aware of the remarkable abilities of even the youngest infants, and experience has taught us that babies need consistent, loving, and even playful interaction with one or more primary caregivers. This interaction must go well beyond basic physical care for babies to grow and develop to their full potential. We have also learned that infants and toddlers are far from passive recipients of care; they actively influence their caregivers and shape the kind of attention they receive (Lewis & Rosenblum, 1974; Sameroff, 1982).

TRENDS IN EARLY INTERVENTION

As our perceptions of infants changed, we developed a belief in the importance of early experience for later development. We began to emphasize the importance of stimulation for both normal and impaired infants.

Changes in our perception of infant and toddler abilities and needs brought changes in public attitudes and policies toward early education. The value of early, regular education had been the focus of some interest since at least the turn of the century with proponents of early education, such as Maria Montessori, demonstrating the efficacy of programs for both normal and retarded or disadvantaged children. The Kennedy era's war on poverty made early education a public policy issue. Compensatory education programs, exemplified by the Head Start programs that began in the 1960s and continue today, were instituted in a belief that educational experiences beginning at three years of age could enhance "disadvantaged" children's ability to do well in school. The overall effects of these programs have been judged to be very favorable (Cooper, 1990) and they have provided the groundwork for even earlier intervention for both normal and impaired children.

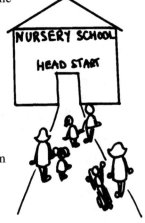

More recently, a shift of public interest away from treatment of existing problems and toward prevention of problems and disabilities has provided support for early intervention. It is generally believed that some of the problems of preschool intervention programs can be solved by intervening earlier. Public awareness of the benefits of providing therapeutic input before the traditional preschool years is increasing. Many programs now serve handicapped (now more frequently called children with disabilities) or at-risk children from birth on.

Fortunately, with the trend toward earlier and earlier intervention has come an awareness of the importance of making room for the infants' and toddlers' families in the therapeutic process. First, parents were included in program offerings; more recently, whole families and their needs have been considered.

Public policy concerning early education and intervention has reflected these changes in attitude. In 1968, P.L. 90-538, the Handicapped Children Early Education Assistance Act, was passed to provide model demonstration centers in which programs addressed the intellectual, physical, social, and emotional development of young, handicapped children. The centers were to provide services to children and their families and training for professionals to work with the children (Rossetti, 1986). P.L. 94-142 and P.L. 99-457, both of which were discussed in earlier chapters, were passed in 1975 and 1986, respectively. These laws provide guidelines and some funds for programming for infants and toddlers who need special input in order to have the best chance to develop to their full potential.

Another influence on the changing programs for young children is the theoretical basis for intervention. As theories of how children learn to talk change, so do our beliefs as to how to help children learn to talk. In the past 40 years we have gone from an emphasis on stimulus and response to concerns with improving cognitive processing and on to enhancing parent-child interactions, in response to the shifts in currently popular theories.

Programs that have been organized to provide early intervention services have reflected all of these changes. Trends in early intervention programming have evolved over the years. Early programs emphasized "enrichment" and "infant stimulation," and often excluded parents from participation in the name of providing an organized regimen of prescribed input. Unfortunately, these initial efforts frequently overlooked basic information on normal development in their zeal to provide stimulation, with the outcome that some infants were actually overstimulated (Zelle, 1976). Early programs were sometimes based on a rigid curriculum which was followed for all children in the program. This emphasis on a set curriculum and "teaching" often ignored the individual needs of a particular child and his or her caregivers (Healy et al., 1985).

The "developmental model" espoused by some programs in which developmental scales dictated the content and sequence of the intervention also had some problems. Like the curriculum based program, this model failed to consider the particular needs of the child and the family and sometimes led to a focus on unimportant behaviors in treatment (Healy et al., 1985).

After attempting to use a number of different approaches in early intervention, practitioners have recognized the value of an individualized, family-centered approach. Fortunately, this is the approach required by P.L. 99-457 (see Chapter 4 for a summary of the requirements of this law).

FAMILY INVOLVEMENT

Current views of best practices in early intervention, such as the approach required by P.L. 99-457, emphasize the importance of family involvement. This involvement goes beyond a relationship in which the professionals are the experts and the families are told what they must do to help their at-risk or impaired member. As Barnard (1984) stated, we must ". . . work with families as a partnership in which we are consultants, but the families are in charge" (p. 4).

The treatment model that has evolved, and which appears to be most appropriate, is one which is family-centered and systems-based. A family-centered approach is one in which the family, not just the child with a communication problem, is the focus of treatment (see Chapter 4). The family's needs and strengths as they relate to the child's communication disorder, and the family's ability to provide for the development of its members, are the focus of intervention. All members of the family may participate in some phase(s) of treatment and all may receive services if that is the best way to facilitate the development of the child.

The systems-based model recognizes that the child is part of a dynamic system made up of individual units (people) who are in ever-changing balance with one another. If one unit of the system shifts or changes, the system will be out of balance until the other portions of the system adjust to the variation in that unit. Family-centered, systems-based treatment can be implemented within the various service delivery paradigms (e.g., home-based, center-based, etc.). A transdisciplinary team approach may be the most efficient model to use, either with or without family members functioning as the team members who implement treatment procedures.

While there is now evidence that family members often function well as intervention agents (Kilburg, 1985; Rees, 1984), there is also some concern that professionals who expect parents to play the role of primary therapists for their child may be expecting too much (McCormick & Schiefelbusch, 1990). Parents may already be overburdened with tasks to do and roles to play; other family members may need the time and attention that would be spent on providing direct treatment for a special-needs child. Strengthening the family system by helping the parents to attend to the needs of all members may ultimately have a more beneficial effect for the child client than having parents involved in time-consuming treatment procedures (McCormick & Schiefelbusch, 1990). As McCormick and Schiefelbusch (1990) state,

> The issue is whether it could be detrimental to family interactions and the stability of the family system for professionals to ask parents to be home teachers. The increased stress and time demands associated with caring for their special-needs child may dictate against parents assuming expanded training roles. (p. 284)

This does not mean that family involvement may have negative consequences for the family system. Involvement in which members maintain their family roles (parents play the role of parents, sisters maintain their stance as sisters) but also provide facilitative interactions for the at-risk or impaired infant or toddler within the context of their day-to-day activities would seem to be possible in most families. This form of family involvement, referred to as "facilitative parenting," will be discussed later in this chapter.

In addition, family members may become involved in treatment at different levels. Alexander, Kroth, Simpson, and Poppelreiter (1982) have identified four levels at which parents can become involved in their child's programming:

1. awareness level—parents are made aware of the child's goals, procedures, and progress
2. knowledge and information level—parents receive specific and extensive information about the child's program
3. meaningful exchanges and interaction level—family members participate in some program-related activities, perhaps by reporting on generalization of skills
4. skill acquisition and training level—family members are directly involved in therapeutic programming for the child.

Among our most important rationales for helping families to become involved in treatment of the communication-disordered or at-risk infant or toddler is the idea that playing a more or less active role in activities, which prevent or remediate problems, helps to "empower" the family and counteracts feelings of helplessness. The level of involvement that will bring about this feeling of empowerment depends on the family. Different families will benefit maximally from different levels of involvement. As stated by McCormick and Schiefelbusch (1990),

> . . . parent involvement (or uninvolvement) is determined by many factors which are not under the immediate control of either professionals or parents. The type and degree of the child's exceptionality, the social and cultural values of the parents, and the strategies they use to cope with problems will all contribute, not only to their needs but also to their participation in their child's programming. (p. 284)

In addition to allowing parents and other family members to become involved at the level they find most comfortable, clinicians must also allow for changes in the family's level of involvement (M. Briggs, May 1991, personal communication). Family members may need or be able to move from one level of involvement to another depending upon other life factors and time demands. Clinicians who can allow or encourage this kind of flexibility may find parents more eager to become involved in treatment.

Families from some cultural backgrounds may be less interested in involvement in treatment than others. Also, some family system characteristics (e.g., family cohesion and adaptability) are likely to influence a family's willingness and ability to participate. And chaotic or dysfunctional families may be hard pressed to become involved in a meaningful way. Whatever the family's apparent circumstance, cultural background, or economic situation, the clinician would be well advised not to make any assumptions about the family's willingness or ability to be involved in treatment without exploring the topic with the family itself.

Models of Involvement/Roles for Family Members

There are many different ways for family members to become involved in communication focused treatment for the infant or toddler. There are also many ways for their interactions with professionals to develop. For example, family members can participate as change agents, take part in parent/family education efforts, or in parent/family support programs. Whatever their level of involvement or model of participation, parents and other family members play various roles in the treatment process.

Turnbull and Turnbull (1986) outline eight historic and current roles of parents of handicapped children. Parents have been seen as:

1. the problem source, the people who created the handicapped child or the conditions that lead to the child's deficit
2. organization members, members of organizations such as the Association for Retarded Citizens, promoting services for handicapped children
3. service developers, active participants in developing services when they are not available
4. recipients of professional decisions
5. learners and teachers, as with programs such as Head Start in which parents were taught to teach their children
6. political advocates, advocating at the local, state, and national levels for improved services and favorable public policy
7. educational decision makers, with P.L. 94-142 and P.L. 99-457 parents have begun to participate in the decisions regarding their childrens' treatment
8. family members, now being recognized as their most important role as units in the family system.

Several of these possible roles can be classified as roles in which the family members act as "change agents," carrying out activities that result in changes in conditions or behaviors that affect their at-risk or impaired family member. There are many ways that parents or other family members can actively participate in changing child behaviors and/or the environment. We have come to think of parents in early intervention programs as intervenors or "substitute therapists" who have been taught to use behavior modification techniques to "teach" their children various tasks. While this is still a possible role for parents to play, it is not the only way for them to effect changes.

Parents who are active as advocates, promoting favorable legislation, may have an equal or greater effect on a child's (or many children's) progress. Also, many parents who have not acted as their child's substitute therapist have played the role of carry-over or generalization agents, attempting to help their child make the difficult transfer of skills from the treatment situation to everyday life.

When parents do play the role of primary or ancillary therapists, actively participating in the child's treatment, it is now less likely that they will be implementing a strict behavioral program. Programs for infants and toddlers have evolved as we have tried a variety of treatment models and methods. The newer approaches, which are more consistent with normal development, allow for more flexibility. With some approaches, the parents can provide important input to the language-learning process without forsaking their role as parents or taking on the time commitment of making special times in each day for "speech lessons." I call this taking on the role of "facilitative parent." Rather than donning a therapist hat and doing special lessons just as the speech-language pathologist showed them, parents can continue carrying out their usual routines with their child. As they complete their usual caregiving and/or play routines, they can be providing language input and responses that are specially tailored to promote language learning in their child. They can do this by learning and using language facilitation techniques that are suggested by a consulting speech-language pathologist. We will consider this role for parents further when we discuss the natural/incidental method of treatment.

TREATMENT MODELS

Two primary models of treatment are used to promote language development with the birth to three population today—natural/incidental language treatment and behavioral treatment/direct teaching programs. Both of these approaches have evolved from earlier programs (Bricker & Carlson, 1981), and have been shown to be effective ways of facilitating language development (McCormick & Schiefelbusch, 1990; Warren & Kaiser, 1986).

An important condition for language learning is the ability of the caregiver and the child to attend to the same object or event as the caregiver talks about that referent. This joint reference makes it possible for the child to link up the verbal symbols used with the appropriate object or event and for language to be meaningful. It follows that in order to promote language development, any program must have some way of establishing and maintaining joint reference with a child.

The next section describes the natural/incidental language treatment (N/ILT) and the behavioral treatment/direct teaching (BT/DT) models of language intervention. It also differentiates these models based on their approach to establishing joint reference.

Natural/Incidental Language Treatment

N/ILT has been called by many different names by various authors who have described it in the literature. It has been called incidental language teaching (Warren & Kaiser, 1986), milieu teaching (Hart & Rogers-Warren, 1978), transactional training (McLean & Snyder-McLean, 1978), child-oriented therapy (Fey, 1986), and naturalistic teaching (McCormick & Schiefelbusch, 1990). All of these variations have certain characteristics in common. According to Warren and Kaiser (1986), all of these approaches are connected by the common ideas:

> (a) that language and communication skills should be taught in the child's natural environment, (b) in conversational contexts, (c) utilizing a dispersed trials training approach that (d) emphasizes following the child's attentional lead, and (e) using functional reinforcers indicated by child requests and attention. . . . Incidental teaching as language intervention involves (a) arranging the environment to increase the likelihood that the child will initiate to the adult and, thus, will provide incidences for teaching; (b) selecting language targets appropriate for the child's skill level, interest, and the opportunities the environment provides; (c) responding to the child's initiations with requests for elaborated language resembling the targeted forms; and (d) reinforcing the child's communicative attempts as well as use of specific forms with attention and access to the objects in which the child has expressed an interest. (p. 291)

This form of language intervention is based largely on the pragmatic and interactionist theories of language development and on information from studies of facilitative language input in the process of normal language acquisition. Because it uses natural interaction in the child's normal environment as the setting for treatment, it is especially appropriate for home-based programs and for use by family members.

In N/ILT, joint attention of the child and adult to an object or event is established by having the adult follow the child's lead. In other words, the adult simply attends to what the child is attending to and provides language input on that topic. This makes it an especially good technique to use even with young infants.

Behavioral Treatment/Direct Teaching Model

Like N/ILT, BT/DT has been referred to by many names such as the didactic approach (Kaiser & Warren, 1988), the trainer-oriented approach (Fey, 1986), and direct teaching (McCormick & Schiefelbusch, 1990). This approach is considered to be more structured than N/ILT and "emphasizes selection of precise, measurable objectives and delineation of explicit and direct instructions and criteria" (McCormick & Schiefelbusch, 1990, p. 191). Correct responses from the child are differentially reinforced, progress is formally monitored, the training environment is structured to elicit attention, and skills to be trained are identified by task analysis (McCormick & Schiefelbusch, 1990).

BT/DT is based on the behavioral theory of language acquisition, but it has been modified over the years to incorporate interactionist ideas. Still, its emphasis is on the form of language, rather than language function.

Because BT/DT is a structured approach with materials and procedures set by the clinician, joint attention must be established by training the child to attend to what the adult is interested in. As discussed in Chapter 7, such attention to adult-selected stimuli is difficult for children less than 18 months of age.

In practice, N/ILT and BT/DT programs are seldom purely naturalistic or behavioral; each often has characteristics of the other, and some programs consciously combine elements of both. Table 9-1 contains a comparison of the two approaches.

TREATMENT METHODS/STRATEGIES

The treatment methods or strategies that will be best suited to a specific child and family will depend upon the characteristics, history, strengths, and needs of the individuals involved. The setting in which treatment is to take place (e.g., center or home) will also play a role in deciding on the methods to be used. The process of assessing the family in general and as a context for language learning will provide important information concerning which methods will be most effective. Assessing the child's communication abilities and establishing treatment goals and objectives with input from all team members, including the

Table 9-1 Comparison of Direct Teaching and Naturalistic Teaching

Factors	Directive Teaching	Naturalistic Teaching
Teaching focus	Emphasis on use of developmentally appropriate language forms and structures (vocabulary, syntax and/or morphology).	Emphasis on increasing successful and functional communication (e.g., requesting). Emphasis on arranging opportunities for child to talk about interesting and desired stimuli and wants. Emphasis on establishing contiguity between the child's attention to an object or event and the label.
Direction of instructional exchanges	Adult-initiated exchanges outnumber child-initiated exchanges. Child always expected to respond.	Child-initiated interactions outnumber adult-initiated exchanges. Adult follows child's lead.
Teaching context and/or locus	Therapy or clinic room or other location isolated from ongoing and naturalistic events/routines.	Natural settings, whenever and wherever instructional opportunities occur.
Nature of instructional exchanges	One-to-one precise and specific teaching trials and sessions. Heavy reliance on massed trial training formats. Use of shaping, fading, imitation, and differential reinforcement.	Child's initiations responded to with expansions and requests for more sophisticated utterances. Instruction similar to that which occurs in caregiver-child dyadic exchanges. Use of prompting and modeling but loose stimulus control.
Reinforcement	High ratio of differential reinforcement for appropriate use of targeted forms and structures.	Child's communicative efforts rewarded by attention and receipt of desired objects, actions, and/or events. Functional consequences—e.g., control of the environment, continued interactions, and achievement of communicative intentions.
Generalization	Planned and trained.	Training in natural contexts during ongoing events, so no special planning/training for generalization.

Source: From *Early Language Intervention,* 2nd ed., (p. 195) by L. McCormick and R. Schiefelbusch, 1990, Columbus, OH: Merrill Publishing Company. Copyright 1990 by Merrill Publishing Company. Reprinted by permission.

family, will also help the clinician to choose the strategies best suited to preventive intervention for a particular child.

In this chapter, emphasis will be placed on N/ILT because of its special usefulness in family-centered intervention. BT/DT will be covered briefly.

Natural/Incidental Treatment Methods

When N/ILT is the model of choice for a particular family, the treatment methods which will be most effective for a specific child can be selected after careful review of the IFSP. Working from the statements of desired outcomes, and using information from the assessment of the family as a context for language learning and of the child's communication skills, specific treatment objectives are written. Individual planning is particularly important if N/ILT is to be effective.

A number of strategies are particularly important to implementation of a N/ILT program. These strategies are adapted from Hart and Rogers-Warren (1978), Warren and Kaiser (1986), Fey (1986), and McCormick and Schiefelbusch (1990). The strategies include:

1. choosing target behaviors that are developmentally appropriate and functional for the child and family
2. arranging the environment to increase the probability that the child will initiate communicative interaction using the target behaviors
3. carefully and consistently following the child's lead in play and communication topics and waiting for the child to initiate interaction
4. "loading" the communicative environment to model the target behaviors using self- and parallel-talk and to respond to the child's communicative behaviors with language-facilitating behaviors
5. providing natural reinforcement for communicative attempts, whether or not the child achieves the target behavior. In the following section, each of these strategies will be discussed in detail.

Strategy #1. Choosing target behaviors that are developmentally appropriate and functional for the child and family; specifically, behaviors that get attention, interaction, or desired goods and services for the child, and that are high priority behaviors for the family. Although the choice of objectives was discussed in Chapter 8, some additional comments on the importance of the nature of the specific behaviors which will be targeted (selected as child behaviors to be elicited, encouraged, and/or reinforced) are in order. The behaviors that may be most appropriate as targets for N/ILT can be selected on the basis of what they "get" for the child or the family. They must be chosen for their importance to interaction and child or family functioning, not for their presence on a developmental scale or in a curriculum guide. They must also be behaviors that have a high likelihood of being used spontaneously by the child in response to conditions that can be created in the environment. Further, they may be behaviors that can appropriately be modeled by a clinician or caregiver. For example, one family's high priority target behaviors for its at-risk toddler may include (1) asking for "juice" by approximating that word and (2) verbally 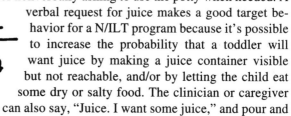 or nonverbally asking to use the potty when needed. A verbal request for juice makes a good target behavior for a N/ILT program because it's possible to increase the probability that a toddler will want juice by making a juice container visible but not reachable, and/or by letting the child eat some dry or salty food. The clinician or caregiver can also say, "Juice. I want some juice," and pour and drink some juice as the child watches. These conditions help to increase the probability that the child will want some juice and will have recently heard an appropriate model for the target behavior.

It is much more difficult to manipulate a child's need to use the potty, even though having the child indicate such a need is an important priority for many families, and this behavior appears as an item on at least one developmental language scale. It is also less appropriate for a clinician to model this behavior for the child.

It should be clear from these examples that careful consideration needs to be given to the choice of target behaviors. This is not to say that other, less easily manipulated behaviors cannot be targeted, but success rates may decline when they are. At least early in treatment, when demonstrable progress is especially important to maintaining motivation, it may be important to choose targets that have a high probability of success.

Strategy #2. Arranging the environment (including the behavior of its human participants) to increase the probability that the child will initiate communicative interaction using target behaviors. This strategy is often one of the creative challenges of this kind of treatment. Once target behaviors are chosen, the clinician asks, "How can we create a need for the child to do that?" or "How can we facilitate the child's use of that behavior (by positioning, availability of stimuli, etc.)?" The environment that we can control has at least two dimensions that we must consider: the physical dimension and the behavioral dimension. In arranging the physical environment there are a number of important considerations. For example, the environment should contain an appropriate amount of stimuli. It should not have so many toys or decorations that the child is tempted to "flit" from thing to thing, attending to so many interesting things that there is no need to comment on or request one especially interesting item. Also, there should be things in the environment that are familiar and comforting to the child (e.g., favorite toys). This is especially important in a clinical or center-based environment.

The environment should also include things that are slightly novel to the child, things that are slightly different from the items that the child sees at home, or familiar things that are used or combined in an unusual way. Children are most likely to talk about things that they can act on, or things that move and change (Nelson, 1973); therefore, our treatment environment must contain things that fit into these categories.

Interesting and desirable items should be evident, but not too readily attainable. A child who can reach and obtain all of the fascinating things he or she sees doesn't need to communicate about them to a caregiver. When things are evident but out of reach, a child must find some way of commenting on or requesting them. Consequently, the environment can be especially tailored to promoting communication if some attractive items are put out of reach.

The "arrangement" of the behavioral environment is just as important as the arrangement of the physical aspects of that environment. General attitudes and behaviors of the people who interact with the child are important considerations in creating an environment that facilitates the use of language and other communicative behaviors. Some of these factors are discussed below. Specific language-facilitating behaviors will be discussed under a later strategy.

People in the child's environment should be attentive and responsive to the child, talking to the child frequently, perhaps by commenting on what the caregiver or child is doing or seeing. This is important behavior even when no specific attempts to stimulate communicative interaction are being made. People should also attempt to create an accepting and warm environment in which interaction can take place. While this is done partially by the arrangement of the physical environment, it is also a product of an attitude that Carl Rogers called "unconditional positive regard." Whatever the child does or doesn't do, he or she is prized and respected as an individual.

One of the most important things people in the child's environment can do is to allow the child the time to initiate some communicative interaction. To do this, people must refrain from being too quick to provide goods or services that they think the child might want or need, while remaining alert to any possible communication from the child. If caregivers can wait for the child to communicate at his or her highest possible level concerning wants and desires, the child will begin to comprehend the power of communication. Without this opportunity, the child will have no need to communicate.

Strategy #3. Carefully and consistently following the child's lead in play and communication topics and waiting for the child to initiate interaction. One factor that has emerged as an important issue in language facilitation is "contingent responding." When the adult's language is contingent upon, or takes its topic from, the child's communication or other behavior, it is apparently more helpful as a language model (Cross, 1984). This stands to reason because when the child and adult both attend to the same event or object, the child can more readily link up the adult's words with their referent. Because it is difficult for an adult to regulate a very young child's attention or to dictate what the child will attend to, this kind of joint attention is most readily attained by the adult paying attention to what the child is interested in. Consequently, contingent responding—the adult following the child's lead in attending to various objects and events and then responding verbally to the child—helps the child to grasp the semantics of the language by helping him or her to link up the words that are used with things in the environment.

Using this strategy takes some practice. Most of us are accustomed to trying to direct children's attention to what we have planned for them or to what we are interested in. We may even have been taught that this is an important part of our clinical job. The edict, "The clinician should always be in control of the session," sounds familiar to most of us, and usually meant that the clinician selected the stimuli that the child should respond to as well as the behaviors that were deemed appropriate as responses. It takes a conscious adjustment in our perception of our role as clinician to feel good about letting the child dictate the focus of attention. Once we have accepted that aspect of N/ILT, we must become skilled at reading the largely nonverbal behavior that tells us what the very young child is interested in. The next step is learning to provide a verbal response to the child that will promote communicative interaction. These responses will be considered under Strategy #4.

Strategy #4. "Loading" the communicative environment to model the target behaviors using self- and parallel-talk in an appropriate way and responding to the child's communicative behaviors with language-facilitating behaviors (e.g., expansions, expatiations) which are semantically contingent on the child's previous action or communication. Our experiences with communication may tell us that the best way to get people to talk to us is to ask questions. Unfortunately, asking questions may not be the best way to encourage verbal interaction with young children. Researchers have identified a number of alternative ways to facilitate talking and to promote language learning (Hubbell, 1977). These techniques include: language modeling using self-talk and parallel-talk; responding techniques called expansion and expatiation; and questioning using open and closed questions.

The first technique, language modeling, is useful with children of any language level, but most useful for children who are not yet talking or are using some words and short sentences. There are two major kinds of language modeling: self-talk and parallel-talk. For self-talk, the adult talks about what he or she is doing, seeing, or thinking in the presence of the child. For example:

> (Adult playing in the sand box with child) "I'm putting sand in this cup. There, it's full. Now I'm pouring the sand on this car. Where's the car? I can't see it. Oh, there it is."

For parallel-talk, the adult talks about what the child is doing, seeing, etc. For example:

> (Same sand box, adult, and child) "Now Bobby's pouring sand on the car. More sand. Where did that car go? Can't see it. Oh, there it is."

Self-talk and parallel-talk allow the child to hear words used and to understand that language is useful and fun. The child isn't asked to respond or imitate.

A second technique for talking with children which focuses on responding to them is called expansion of the child's sentences. This technique is useful with children who are talking but using incomplete sentences. The adult listens to the child's sentence or word, tries to understand the whole idea the child is attempting to communicate, and repeats the child's sentence in a grammatically complete but simple form. This lets the child know that he or she was understood and allows him or her to hear the complete sentence. For example:

> *Child:* "Doggy bark."
> *Adult:* "Yes, the doggy is barking."

This technique is most powerful if it is not used too much. If it's used constantly, the child gets few chances to truly communicate and have someone respond naturally to his or her communication.

A third technique, called expatiation, is concerned with just this kind of natural communication. It is accomplished by simply following the child's lead in a conversation. The adult focuses on what the child says rather than how he or she says it. The adult acknowledges what the child has said and often adds some new information. For example:

> *Child:* "Boy run."
> *Adult:* "Yes, he's in a hurry."

Child: "Go school."
Adult: "I think you're right; here comes his school bus now."

This technique is helpful to any child or adult. It shows that what they say is important and helps them to understand the pleasure of communication.

Another technique involves questioning. There are two major kinds of questions: open questions and closed questions. Open questions are questions that can be answered in a variety of ways and at great length if the child wishes.

"How can I make this work?"
"What do you like to do, Bobby?"
"What did you and Daddy do outside?"

Closed questions can be answered with a short phrase or a one-word answer. Often the adult knows the answers to these questions and uses them to test or display the child's knowledge or verbal ability.

"How many balls are there here?"
"What color is this car?"
"Who is this?"

Children often fail to answer questions like this because they know the asker doesn't really need the information. Open questions are probably most useful for starting conversations with children.

The more a child can be allowed to initiate and direct a conversation, the more he or she will talk, the more practice he or she will get with communicating, and the better he or she will feel about his or her skills as a talker.

Appendix 9-A contains a parent handout based on these language-facilitating behaviors.

Strategy #5. Providing natural reinforcement (e.g., giving requested goods or services) for communicative attempts whether or not they achieve the target behavior. Reinforcement, which is technically any response that follows a behavior and which produces an increase in that behavior, is an important tool for increasing language behavior that was first recognized by the behaviorists. In behavioral treatment, reinforcement is carefully planned and controlled by the clinician. In N/ILT, the nature of the reinforcement is usually not as carefully planned in advance because it is to be determined by the child's communicative behavior. Rather than giving the child an edible reward or verbal praise for each correct production of a target behavior, as might occur in a behavioral program, the N/ILT clinician tries to follow the attempt at communicating with its natural consequence. For example, if the child squeals with delight upon seeing some event, the clinician may focus his or her attention on the same event and agree with the child's assessment by saying something like, "You're right, that dog looks very silly!" If possible, the clinician may cause the event to occur again. Or, if a child requests a certain toy, perhaps by pointing, making eye contact with the clinician, and vocalizing, the clinician will provide the toy for the child as quickly as possible, using the opportunity to model the label for the toy. Even if the behavior being targeted is use of single words and the child is not using words, reinforcement is given for the communicative attempt and paired with the model of a higher level of behavior. If modeling fails to elicit imitation of the word, the pause between the clinician's model and the provision of reinforcement might be increased to allow time for the child to imitate the model, but the requested goods or services should still be provided to reinforce the communication used. They should be provided especially quickly, paired with positive affect such as smiles and head nodding, if the child imitates the word.

These five strategies are useful as guidelines for structuring interactions with children who are at risk for, or have problems with, language learning. Another concept that plays a role in N/ILT is "scaffolding." Scaffolding describes strategies used by parents and other adults to support children's learning of complex tasks or abilities. One primary way that adults provide scaffolding for language learning is with social routines (Snow, 1984). Social routines are sequences of events that occur in the same way over and over. These routines involve language behavior which is repeated in the same way each time the routine is used. The language is always the same and is therefore predictable and relatively easy for the child to learn and participate in. Greetings, courtesies such as saying "please," "thank you," and "excuse me," rhymes, songs, and favorite books are all part of routines that provide scaffolding for language learning. It is usually helpful to include some social routines in which the child can participate in a language program.

Once routines are established, it may be helpful to create a need to communicate by interrupting the routine in some way. McCormick and Schiefelbusch (1990), citing Halle, Albert, and Anderson (1984), suggest three ways to interrupt routines that may elicit comment from young children.

Delay provision of an expected and desired material or event. For example, the typical sequence after the children are seated at the snack table is to pass napkins, pour juice or milk, and then distribute pieces of fruit. One day, after the napkins and juice have been dispensed, the teacher simply waits (with the plate of fruit in hand). When the child (or children) have requested or commented, then she dispenses the treat as expected.

Provide an incomplete set of materials and wait. This is most appropriate for routines such as art or cooking projects. Children are provided with an incomplete set of materials to elicit a protest or request for the missing materials. For this procedure to work, the routine must be inherently reinforcing and it must require a pre-scribed set of materials.

Make "silly" mistakes. For example, calling a child by the wrong name will prompt spontaneous language (a correction). Children are usually quick to respond to absurdities and inappropriate actions. Examples are such silly mistakes as pulling a toothbrush from a purse and pretending to brush one's hair or holding a book upside down. In addition to prompting spontaneous protest, this type of behavior has the added advantage of helping children develop a sense of humor. (p. 240)

These strategies and concepts are the bases for individually tailored N/ILT programs. In addition, the following general ideas and tenets should be kept in mind:

1. Conduct treatment in the child's home environment or in a setting that is as much like the child's home environment as possible including people, toys, etc.
2. Make treatment communication oriented, not a drill.
3. Convey as much acceptance as you can to the child in your words and nonverbal behaviors.
4. Present stimuli in as many sense modalities as possible.
5. Try to communicate to very young children, "You can have an effect on your environment. You can make something happen."
6. Interpret behaviors as communicative behaviors and they will become communicative behaviors. Expect the child to communicate.
7. Provide a language model that relates to the "here and now" and is tailored to the child's language level and target behaviors using self- and parallel-talk.
8. Keep your speech rate fairly slow (under 200 syllables per minute).
9. Give the child choices whenever possible.
10. Take turns, allowing plenty of time for the child to organize his or her behavior for a turn.

Most of these treatment strategies can easily be adapted to fit the family's ethnic background or culture. Some of the strategies (e.g., #3, following the child's lead in play and communication) or the suggested language facilitation techniques may not be typical language teaching strategies for some cultures. As noted in other sections of the book, it is always wise to become familiar with the specific cultural characteristics and values of the families with whom you are working and to adopt as many of their strategies as possible.

Play As a Treatment Tool

One of the powerful tools that we can use in N/ILT is play. Play is a natural context for language learning because it provides the motivation of having fun as well as opportunities for modeling and responding to communication that is part of the play situation.

Not everything that involves toys is play. It is sometimes tempting to assume that any activity that uses dolls, balls, blocks, or puppets is intrinsically motivating to children because it is play. Play isn't defined by the materials used but by the attitude and freedom with which those materials are employed. Activities that are truly playful are pleasureable, have no conscious extrinsic goals, are spontaneous and voluntary, involve active participation, and can be distinguished in some way from what is not play (Garvey, 1977).

Various kinds of play may be used as a context for N/ILT with infants and toddlers. Sensorimotor play, symbolic or representational play, motor play, parallel play, play with objects, play with language, and dramatic play are all part of the experience of normal infants and toddlers.

Play helps the child to learn about the environment through assimilation (changing things to fit your schema) and accomodation (changing your schema to fit environmental pressures). It also provides opportunities for children to learn about social interaction as they adapt to others' needs and desires and learn social rules and roles in play. Play and language appear to have a common cognitive base because their development is parallel in many ways (Terrell et al., 1984).

Not all toys are equally useful for language-promoting activities. Toys that require cooperation and interaction or that allow the child to recreate social situations may be the best for inclusion in early intervention programs. Parten (1971) suggested that toys such as a house and dolls, kiddie cars, clay, blocks, scissors and paper, sand trays, paints, swings, beads, and trains may have the greatest potential for promoting social participation. Food-related toys such as dishes, cups, and flatware are also useful in interactive play. Wanska et al. (1986) found that children's topic performance differed depending upon the play materials used, with miniature hospital toys creating more interactive play than Legos.

The stategies, concepts, and tenets employed to use play in the treatment situation are the same as those discussed above. To plan play-oriented N/ILT, start with the assessment information and consider where the child is developmentally in terms of play and communication. Then decide what the next appropriate level for communication development is and how children normally use play to get to that next level. Devise treatment goals, objectives, and procedures that use the child's current play skills to move him or her to the next level of communication ability.

The next section discusses a somewhat different orientation toward language treatment—behavioral treatment or direct teaching methods.

Behavioral Treatment/Direct Teaching Methods

The teaching methods or strategies that are employed in BT/DT programs have been developed and used in behavioral programs for many years and with many different populations. Although the strategies are used in a conscious and systematic way in BT/DT programs (McCormick & Schiefelbusch, 1990), they are approaches that occur on a less formal level in all human interaction. The strategies most commonly used in behavioral or direct teaching programs include: (1) controlled presentation of stimuli and modeling; (2) prompting; (3) shaping; (4) specification of responses which are considered to be correct; (5) reinforcement of correct responses; and (6) generalization.

Strategy #1. Controlled presentation of stimuli and modeling. Because behaviorally oriented programs select and specify the objects and events that are used in teaching procedures, they often specify how those stimuli are to be presented to the child. In some programs, the clinician's presentation of stimuli is scripted (e.g., Gray & Ryan, 1973) and is to be given in a precise manner. Modeling is the presentation of an example of the desired behavior which the child is to 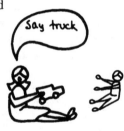 imitate. In behavioral programs, the model is often accompanied by an instruction to, "Say ___." This instruction is called a "mand," and it is a command or request for a certain behavior.

The presentation of stimuli is especially important in behavioral programs because of the issue of joint attention which was discussed earlier. Only with careful and sensitive presentation techniques can the very young child's attention be directed to an object or event of the clinician's choice.

Strategy #2. Prompting. When an imitative response is not readily given following the presentation of the stimulus, prompting may be used. A prompt is a behavior that assists and supports a response. It may be a verbal or vocal prompt that gives the child the first sound in the target word that is the correct response, or it may be a physical prompt, such as pointing toward the object that has been requested or moving the child's hand in that direction.

Strategy #3. Shaping. Shaping is used when the child is not yet able to produce the correct response. The correct response is shaped by reinforcing either component parts of a complex response or closer and closer approximations of a difficult response (Fey, 1986; McCormick & Schiefelbusch, 1990).

Strategy #4. Specification of responses that are considered to be correct. With behavioral programming, only those responses that are considered correct are reinforced and allow for progression in the program. Therefore, the exact characteristics of a correct response must be specified.

Strategy #5. Reinforcement. Positive reinforcement occurs when an event that follows a response serves to strengthen or increase the frequency of that response. When a clinician identifies a positive reinforcer, he or she gains an important tool for increasing desired behaviors. Many different events—from receiving a favorite food to eat, to getting a smile or a touch or a requested turn on the swing—act as reinforcers. Most clinicians find that reinforcers that are natural consequences of the desired behavior, such as being granted a requested turn, are most effective in language programs.

Strategy #6. Generalization. If we had to teach a child to respond with a given behavior to every situation where that response was appropriate, we would have an impossible task before us. Fortunately, many responses generalize to other, similar situations without formal instruction, especially when they have been learned under natural conditions. Only when a response has generalized to untaught situations can we consider it to be truly learned and under the child's control. One of the primary criticisms of behavioral approaches is that learned responses often fail to generalize to other situations without specific generalization training. Consequently, elaborate procedures have been designed to generalize or carry-over learned behaviors to other situations.

These two treatment methods, N/ILT and BT/DT, are sometimes combined in one child's program or in the treatment approach adopted by an institution. Behavioral strategies, such as prompting and shaping, can complement N/ILT when they are used in the spirit of the strategies and tenets of that approach.

One example of a program that combines behavioral and natural strategies is described by Fitzgerald and Karnes (1987). They report that "an ecological approach to language intervention has begun to evolve that uses behavioral techniques to facilitate the acquisition of developmentally appropriate communication skills within the context of parent-child interactions in daily teaching and caregiving environments" (p. 32). This and similar programs may combine the best features of both approaches for use with some children and families.

In the next section ways to use N/ILT in the family context are considered as well as focusing on strategies for helping family members to use N/ILT strategies and to become facilitative parents.

Helping Families To Facilitate Communication Development

When family members are to be involved in treatment, either as ancillary clinicians or facilitative parents, they need to be provided with opportunities to learn to use the teaching and/or facilitation techniques under positive and supportive conditions that are consistent with principles of adult learning. Adults tend to learn best by active participation that involves problem solving (Anderson, Beckett, Chitwood, Hayden, & Hitz, 1990). They don't become skilled users of intervention techniques just by watching clinicians work with their child (Culatta & Horn, 1981).

There are a number of techniques that can be used to introduce family members to language treatment and facilitation. Techniques that have been reported in the literature include both group and individual education approaches as well as methods that are more like consultation to the family by the speech-language pathologist. Some approaches involve group instruction in behavior management, consisting primarily of lecture and discussion (e.g., Eyberg & Matarazzo, 1980). Others provide for viewing of a self-instructional video program. Still others provide individual instruction involving some combination of presentations of information on strategies, observation of treatment, parent participation with the clinician in treatment, discussion of strategies, practice of the strategies with the child while being observed by the clinician, discussion of parent use of the strategies, parent practice of the strategies at home with the child, measurement of child progress, and feedback to the parent on the child's progress (Culatta & Horn, 1981).

To help parents learn to use language-facilitation techniques in daily life situations with their child, systematic, individual instruction in language facilitation within the context of natural interaction has been used. This instruction often includes the use of verbally presented information on strategies, written information, videotaped information, demonstration, practice, feedback, and further practice (e.g., MacDonald, 1989; MacDonald & Gillette, 1984).

A very useful and innovative addition to this kind of parent/family education is the use of videotaped practice and feedback. Videotaping parents in interaction with their children prior to treatment and as they practice techniques they have studied and/or observed and playing all or part of these videos for parents has been shown to be an effective aid to helping families change interactive behaviors (Guitar, Kopff, Kilburg, & Conway, 1981; Kilburg, 1985; Girolametto, Greenberg, & Manolson, 1986; McDade & Simpson, 1984; McDade & Varnedoe, 1987).

The following sequence of instruction, adapted from clinical practice and the approaches cited above, is one comprehensive approach to helping families to facilitate communication development in at-risk or language-deficient infants and toddlers.

1. Evaluate videotaped parent-child interaction following the suggestions given in Chapter 6.

2. Verbally present information on language-facilitation techniques tailored to the culture and education level of the family.

3. Give the same information in a written form so that it can be read and shared with other family members. (See the parent handout in Appendix 9-A for an example; also see *Hanen Parent Program Guidebooks* [Manolson, 1985] and MacDonald [1989].)

4. Arrange to view professionally prepared instructional videos that illustrate language-facilitation techniques with family members or loan them copies to be viewed at home. Examples of useful videos include the Hanen Early Language Resource Centre videos, *Oh Say What They See,* and MacDonald's (1989) *Introduction to the ECO Program.*

5. View portions of the original assessment video with the parents looking for examples of behaviors that work with their child. The clinician may select portions of these tapes prior to the session with the family. The clinician takes the lead in pointing out positive parent behaviors. Parents should be allowed to take the lead concerning behaviors that are not as facilitative. That is, don't use this as an opportunity to call parents' attention to their negative behaviors. If they point out instances when they could have used facilitative techniques and did not, acknowledge their statements (e.g., "Yes, that would have been a good place to use parallel-talk and follow your child's lead.") and move on.

6. The parents and clinician can then decide on facilitative behaviors to increase or begin using (e.g., following the child's lead, self-talk, parallel-talk, expansions).

7. Parents can first try these behaviors by role playing them with each other or with the clinician.

8. Once they understand the use of the behaviors, parents can practice them one at a time in videotaped play interaction with their child.

9. In the next session with the clinician, the parents and clinician can view all or clinician-selected portions of the video from the last session, again

emphasizing behaviors that work with their child. Parents can critique their own use of techniques and discuss their progress with the clinician.

10. The parents again practice behaviors in videotaped interaction.

11. Between sessions, parents can practice the facilitative behaviors with their child.

12. The clinician assesses parent and child progress from the videotaped interaction.

Steps 9, 10, 11, and 12 are repeated until parents and clinician feel comfortable with mastery of techniques and the child is progressing well. If the child's communication behavior does not change, techniques are reassessed by the parents and clinician, looking for possible reasons for lack of progress and alternative strategies to use.

In this approach, video plays an important role in helping parents to learn about techniques and to master their use. Parents quickly see how the facilitative techniques work with their child and become motivated to use the strategies. The clinician can play the role of consultant to family members who provide facilitative interaction, and family members can experience the pleasure of promoting language growth while still maintaining their roles as parents, siblings, etc.

CONCLUSION

This chapter has addressed many aspects of family-centered early intervention. The next chapter considers strategies for evaluating family-centered programs.

Appendix 9-A

Parent Handout

TALKING WITH CHILDREN

One of the most important things we do to help our children to learn language is to talk with them. That sounds simple, but I've learned that it's not as simple as it sounds. The hard part is knowing how to talk with a child in ways that are most helpful for language learning. There are some ways that work better than others. I think it's important that parents as well as professionals learn and use these techniques with children. Children not only spend more time with parents, but are also constantly communicating with and learning from their parents. Parents are powerful and important teachers! Here are some suggestions for talking with children:

1. The first technique is called language modeling. It is useful with children of any language level, but most useful for children who are not yet talking or are using some words and short sentences. An adult provides a helpful language model for a child when he or she uses simple, complete sentences. There are two major kinds of language modeling: self-talk and parallel-talk.

For self-talk, you, the parent, talk about what you are doing, seeing, or thinking in the presence of the child. For example:

> (Adult playing in the sand box with child) "I'm putting sand in this cup. There, it's full. Now I'm pouring the sand on this car. Where's the car? I can't see it. Oh, there it is."

For parallel-talk the adult talks about what the child is doing, seeing, etc. For example:

> (Same sand box, adult, and child) "Now Bobby's pouring sand on the car. More sand. Where did that car go? Can't see it. Oh, there it is."

Self-talk and parallel-talk allow the child to hear words used and to understand that language is useful and fun—it adds something nice to the play. The child isn't asked to respond or imitate. If he or she does imitate your words or talk with you, that's wonderful, but it's not required.

2. A second technique for talking with children is called expansion of the child's sentences. This technique is very useful with children who are talking, but using incomplete sentences. The adult listens to the child's sentence or word, tries to understand the whole idea the child is trying to express, and then repeats the child's sentence in a grammatically complete but simple form. This lets the child know that you understood what he or she said and allows him or her to hear the complete sentence. For example:

Child: "Doggy bark."
Adult: "Yes, the doggy is barking."

This technique is most powerful if you don't use it too much. If it's used constantly, the child never gets a chance to truly communicate and have some respond naturally to his communication.

3. A third suggestion for talking with children is concerned with just this kind of natural communication. It's technical name is expatiation, but it is simply following the child's lead in a conversation. The adult focuses on what the child says rather than how he or she says it. The adult acknowledges what the child has said and often adds some new information:

Child: "Boy run."
Adult: "Yes, he's in a hurry."
Child: "Go school."
Adult: "I think you're right; here comes his school bus now."

This technique is helpful to any child or adult. It shows that what they say is important to you and helps them to understand the pleasure of communication.

4. Another way that we often talk with children involves questioning. There are two major kinds of questions: open questions and closed questions. Open questions are questions that can be answered in a variety of ways and at great length if the child wishes, such as

"How can I make this work?"
"What do you like to do, Bobby?"
"What did you and Daddy do outside?"

Closed questions can be answered with a short phrase or one-word answer. Often the adult knows the answers to these questions and uses them to test or display the child's knowledge or verbal ability. For example:

"How many balls are there here?"
"What color is this car?"
"Who is this?"

Children often fail to answer questions like this because they know the asker doesn't really need the information.

Questions are valuable ways of getting information, but they should probably be used sparingly. Unfortunately, the child's most common answer to a question is, "I don't know." If you want to start a conversation with a child with a question, open questions are probably most useful.

Other techniques that people use with children include: correcting the child's speech, using open-ended sentences so that the child will "fill in the blank," and asking the child to imitate your speech. These techniques are useful when used carefully, but they must be used with caution. They give the child little chance to really communicate and can, if used too much, give him or her a real feeling of failure.

Generally, language modeling, expansion, and natural communication are most useful to the child and are therefore the best teaching tools. Also, the more the child can be allowed to initiate and direct a conversation, the more s/he will talk, the more practice s/he will get with communicating, and the better s/he will feel about his or her skills as a talker. You can be most helpful by responding to what your child says and staying on the topic s/he chooses.

These suggestions are all taken from studies of parents talking with children, so I wouldn't be surprised if you already do many of them. You might try to become aware of the techniques you use when you talk with your child. If you use some more than others, try some of the techniques you don't use to see how they work with your child.

It's not necessary to have a special "speech session" with your child to do these things. All of these techniques can fit in with your everyday activities and interactions with your child.

One last thought. Feeling good about ourselves probably increases talking and general positive behavior more than anything. The more praise, encouragement, and other forms of "positive feedback" you can give your child, the more likely he or she is to communicate comfortably with everyone.

Appendix 9-B

Family-Centered Treatment Plan for the C. Family

A family-centered treatment plan can be developed using the information in Chapters 8 and 9. For Todd, who also served as an example in the appendices of Chapters 6 and 7, the following treatment plan was developed in collaboration with Mrs. C. This example is not intended as a model for a legal document, but as a source of information on treatment planning for this child.

Child's Name: Todd C.   Date: 7/10/90
Birthdate: 10/15/87   Age: 33 months

Developmental Levels

Fine Motor: Age appropriate   Gross Motor: Age appropriate
Cognitive: Age appropriate   Social/Emotional: Age appropriate
Self Help: Age appropriate
Language (Receptive): 32 months
(Expressive): 20 months
Vision: Within normal limits
Hearing: Within normal limits

Family Members, Social Supports (Primary Family Roles)

Mrs. C: primary caregiver, part-time breadwinner, homemaker.
Mr. C: breadwinner, home-repairs, occasional caregiver.
Katie: student, playmate for Todd.
Grandmother and Grandfather C: occasional caregivers, social support for parents.

Family and Child Strengths and Needs

Mrs. C. is very concerned about her children's development and wants to do everything possible to help them to be ready for school. She has time to be involved in Todd's treatment and is eager to participate. Mr. C, with Mrs. C's part-time help, provides well financially for the family's needs for food, shelter, etc.

Mrs. C wants Todd to be able to ask for things that he wants and to answer questions so that people can understand him. She wants him to talk clearly and smoothly, and to know colors, numbers, letters, etc., before he goes to school. She wants to make sure that she is doing everything she can to help Todd's development. She feels that she needs help talking with her husband and parents-in-law about Todd's speech and language.

Todd seems to have a strong attachment to his mother. He is shy with other children, and dependent upon his mother to interpret his verbal communication to others.

Desired Outcomes, Treatment Objectives, Strategies, Criteria, and Timelines

Outcome #1
Todd will increase his expressive language abilities so that he can make requests, answer questions, talk clearly, and use basic concepts at an age-appropriate level.

Objective A. Todd will use intelligible, fluent, three- to four-word utterances (MLU = > 3.0) to request and respond during free play with a familiar caregiver by 1/10/91.

Strategies:

1. Adults interacting with Todd will:
   - follow his lead in play and verbal interaction giving semantically related responses
   - use short, simple sentences
   - use fairly slow speech with pauses for him to respond or initiate
   - express as much acceptance of Todd's attempts to communicate and appropriate play choices as possible both verbally and nonverbally
2. The home and treatment environment will be arranged to increase the probability that Todd will need to request things that he wants.
3. Adults and older children will model appropriate requests and responses, and use self- and parallel-talk, expansions, etc.

4. Todd will receive natural reinforcers for attempts at communication (e.g., if he requests a certain food, he gets it as a reinforcer when practical).

Objective B. Todd will express an understanding of primary colors, numbers to ten, prepositions, and size during structured play with appropriately colored and sized toys by 1/10/91.

Strategy:

1. Adults and older children will talk about colors of various objects, model counting to ten, use "in, on, and under" during play interactions, and talk about big and little objects, people, etc. Simple games may ask Todd to find a "big one" or something "under the chair," etc., with positive consequences when he is correct. All interactions should remain playful, with no pressure to perform.

Outcome #2

Mrs. C will increase her feelings of confidence about her ability to promote Todd's language development by learning to interact with him in a facilitative way.

Objective C. Mrs. C will learn language-facilitation techniques and use them with Todd, acting as his primary language change agent.

Strategies:

1. Mrs. C will discuss language development and facilitation with the clinician. She will participate in videotaped interaction with Todd and practice selected facilitation techniques. She will later view the tapes with the clinician to see what "works" best, and continue to practice those techniques with Todd.
2. Mrs. C will learn to use all of the strategies discussed under Outcome #1.
3. Mrs. C will be videotaped with Todd periodically to ascertain whether the facilitation techniques and other strategies are working for both of them. Impact on the rest of the family will also be discussed.

Outcome #3

Mrs. C will increase her ability to discuss Todd's language and speech ability by gaining information on language development and facilitation techniques which she can share with her family and by attending (and inviting them to attend) family-centered workshops on parenting children with speech and language problems.

Objective D. Mrs. C will be able to discuss Todd's speech and langauge without feeling "silly."

Strategies:

1. Mrs. C will obtain written information on language development, language problems, and language facilitation to share with her family. This information will be provided or suggested by the clinician by 8/10/90.
2. Mrs. C, Mr. C, and Todd's grandparents will be invited to participate in a series of family-centered workshops on parenting children with speech and language problems with members of other families of children with language disorders by 9/10/90.
3. Mr. C and/or Todd's grandparents and sister will be invited to participate in Todd's treatment sessions whenever Mrs. C wishes to invite them throughout the treatment period.

Criteria: As stated in the objectives.

Timeline: To be reviewed in three months (10/90) and updated in six months (1/91).

This treatment plan was based on Mrs. C's stated priorities and the clinician's beliefs and past experiences. While Objective B under Outcome #1 would not have been one of the clinician's highest priorities, she helped to develop an objective and strategies that fulfilled both Mrs. C's desires and the clinician's criteria for age-appropriate treatment goals and strategies by making the strategies play-based and natural rather than drill oriented. This plan uses information from the analysis presented in Appendix 6-A to develop specific strategies for language-facilitation techniques.

THE TREATMENT PROGRAM

A treatment program was designed in which Mrs. C was to act as the primary language change agent. She was to learn to modify her language input and responses to Todd, as outlined in the plan above, so that she could provide a more optimal language-learning environment for him. After learning this in the treatment sessions, she would be able to provide this improved environment during their daily interactions.

Todd and his mother were seen for seven treatment sessions, once weekly. Todd's father and other family members were unable to attend any of the sessions. The format of each treatment session was as follows: Mrs. C and the clinician began by discussing the previous session, progress and events of the intervening week, and theories and information on speech and language development. They then viewed clinician-selected portions of Mrs. C's videotaped interaction with Todd from the previous session. These segments were discussed, often with the clinician pointing out instances of the mother's behaviors that appeared to be especially facilitative of Todd's speech or language output. Todd's communicative behaviors were often singled out for attention when they showed longer word combinations, increased vocabulary use, or new syntactic structures. An attempt was made throughout to emphasize positive behaviors, rather than to criticize less helpful techniques.

During these discussion sessions, Todd played with an assistant in another part of the large treatment room. After discussion of the videotape, two or three of the mother's behaviors which appeared to be especially facilitative of Todd's speech and language output in the previous session were singled out. It was suggested that Mrs. C practice these techniques or target behaviors (e.g., using short sentences, using a slow speech rate) during this session's videotaping and at home during the following week.

Mrs. C and Todd were then videotaped in 15 minutes of play-oriented interaction. After the videotaping, the target behaviors were quickly reviewed and plans were made for the next treatment sessions. Each treatment session lasted approximately 50 minutes.

Mrs. C also received handout materials on speech and language development and language facilitation (see Appendix 9-A), and the Bibliography. She participated in a workshop/support group with four other mothers. Her husband and in-laws did not attend any of the sessions.

TREATMENT OUTCOME

Mrs. C proved to be a faithful participant in treatment, never missing a session, and a talented and motivated language facilitator. She learned strategies quickly and credited the videotaped playback with her rapid ability to change. She stated that once she saw what she had been doing she was highly motivated to change. She even suggested that other parents be shown her tapes so that they'd know how important the facilitating techniques were. Original objectives and outcomes are listed below:

Objective A. Todd will use intelligible, fluent, three- to four-word utterances (MLU = > 3.0) to request and respond during free play with a familiar caregiver by 1/10/91.

Todd's MLU went from 1.4 morphemes to 3.29 morphemes. His percent syllables repeated changed from 37.9 to 10.2 percent. The percentage of intelligible utterances went from 40 to 90.4 percent. At the end of treatment Todd used a wide variety of communicative intentions including requests and responses to questions.

Objective B. Todd will express an understanding of primary colors, numbers to ten, prepositions, and size during structured play with appropriately colored and sized toys by 1/10/91.

As Todd's language ability improved, Mrs. C lost interest in this objective. Todd frequently displayed an understanding of these basic concepts.

Objective C. Mrs. C will learn language-facilitation techniques and use them with Todd, acting as his primary language change agent.

Mrs. C's speech and language to Todd changed markedly during treatment. Her MLU went from 5.42 morphemes for the total sample (a difference of 4.02 morphemes from Todd's) to 4.61 morphemes when Todd's was 3.29 (a difference of 1.32 morphemes). Figure 9-B-1 shows how their MLUs related to each other throughout treatment.

Mrs. C's speech rate changed from 350 SPM for the larger sample to 205 SPM. Her percent of semantically related utterances went from 40.9 percent for the larger sample to 92.9 percent, and her percent of accepting responses went from 47.7 percent for the larger sample to 85.7 percent.

A sample of Todd and his mother's interaction during a treatment sessions (see Exhibit 9-B-2) shows how their interaction changed.

Objective D. Mrs. C will be able to discuss Todd's speech and language without feeling "silly."

Mrs. C reported that as Todd's language ability changed, her family began to understand why she had been so concerned, and she felt more comfortable talking with them about it. On many occasions, Mrs. C expressed her satisfaction with her new abilities as a language facilitator and advocate for the techniques she had learned. She clearly felt confident that she had been right to be concerned and to participate in Todd's treatment.

Figure 9-B-1 MLU: Todd and Mother

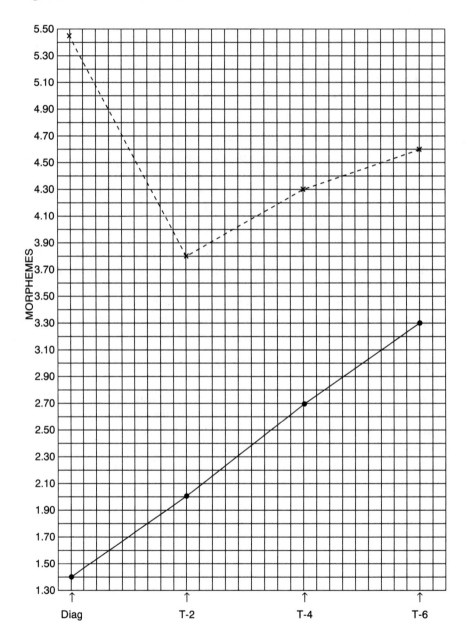

Figure 9-B-2

Child	Nonverbal	Adult
But soap is on my hands	Takes tissue & wipes hands & then counter	
	Watches - attends	1. Soap on your hands again
Counter too		
		2. And the counter, too?
MHM	Throws tissue away	
Go /ɔɪ/ [off] bubbles	Returns to sink	
		3. Go away bubbles
	Dumps bubbles from dish - takes another tissue	4. My goodness
Bubbles on my hand 'gain		
	Laughs	
		5. Okay
Not on /ʌ/ [the] counter		
		6. Not on the counter
	Takes tissue to trash then brings it back - takes jar from shelf puts tissue in & top on - empties in trash	7. Not this time.
? The top on		
		8. Okay, that worked
/bo bʌm bʌm/	Drops "teapot"	
Teapot falls off, too		
		9. The tea fell off, too
	Picks it up	
This on top		
Bubbles on my hands again	Takes another tissue wipes hands & throws away	
	Laughs	10. Bubbles are on your hand again
Dishes		
Dishes		
Dishes		

10

Evaluating Program Effectiveness

One of the most important tasks in early intervention programming is the evaluation of program effectiveness. Program evaluation allows us to find out what works for both a specific child and family and for our clients in general. It allows us to identify any unmet needs of our clients so that we can develop more comprehensive services. It also provides the all-important evidence of efficacy that supports our requests for continued funding.

Despite the importance of the task, it is not an easy one. There are a number of problems inherent in the process of program evaluation that make it difficult to accomplish. Two primary difficulties with research into the efficacy of treatment approaches relate to use of control groups (we cannot, of course, ethically withhold treatment from one group just to prove the validity of our program) and the problem of finding appropriate methods to measure change that can be attributed to the intervention provided by the program (Bailey & Bricker, 1984; Bricker & Carlson, 1981; Fewell & Sandall, 1986). The problem of measurement of change will be discussed in greater detail below.

ISSUES OF PROGRAM EVALUATION

Before program evaluation is begun, a number of issues must be addressed. Bailey and Simeonsson (1988) recommend that we consider the nature, adequacy, and interpretability of information that we gather for an evaluation. Related to the nature of the information to be gathered, Ziggler and Berman (1983) suggest that we must decide (1) who and what should be the focus of the evaluation and (2) how and when the evaluation should be done. Let's look at these issues one at a time.

Who and what should be the focus of the evaluation? There are three potential beneficiaries of family-centered early intervention programs: the child, the parents and other family members, and the community in general (Ziggler & Berman, 1983). Any one or all of these may be the focus of evaluation. We often think of the child and his or her progress toward the desired outcomes—as assessed by various achievement measures—as the primary beneficiary of treatment, but the child is not the only one who may profit. In family-centered treatment we have not only the indirect benefits to the family that often occur in child-centered treatment (e.g., the parents' relationship with one another improves because some of the stress of having an impaired child is relieved when they feel they are providing the treatment the child needs). Because some of the outcomes may target the family, there are also direct benefits related to treatment. Consequently, it is important to focus on measurable changes in the family as well as the child, such as increases in needed information, language-facilitation ability, or availability of support. For both the child and family, those characteristics and behaviors most relevant to the program's goals and objectives should be assessed by some means (Bailey & Simeonsson, 1988).

Another aspect of program evaluation that has received attention in family-centered programs is that of client satisfaction and the actual family centeredness of the program. Even when positive change can be documented for the child and family, those changes, or the program itself, may be less than satisfactory if some aspect(s) of the program is (are) problematic for the families served.

The third possible beneficiary of early intervention programs is the community in which the early intervention services are located, or more specifically, the social institutions in that community. It may be possible to measure changes such as shifts in public awareness of handicapping conditions, strategies for prevention and treatment of disability, acceptance of individual differences, etc., that are attributable to the program's presence in the community.

How and when should programs be evaluated? How to measure changes in variables such as communication ability or social competence in our child clients for program evaluation purposes remains problematic and relates to the adequacy of the information on which we base our evaluation. Fewell and Sandall (1986) discuss the use of various measures to assess progress in young handicapped children. They note that developmental age scores, developmental quotients, and prediction indices which are often used in research on treatment efficacy can give quite different views of treatment progress in the same subjects. These authors note that developmental age scores may inflate the evidence of a positive outcome because they fail to consider the effects of maturity over time. A different issue may arise with the use of developmental quotients that do correct for age differences. If impaired infants' initial scores on these measures are unexpectedly high, which they sometimes are due to insensitivity of the measure to differences in very young children (measures often have very few items at the early age levels), later evaluation on the same measure may be more accurate (often being based on a wider sample of behavior) and evaluate the child at a lower developmental quotient. When this occurs, it appears that the child failed to progress or even lost ground when in fact the difference is due to error of measurement.

A similar problem occurs with prediction analysis when initial scores are high, resulting in unrealistically high predicted post-test scores. There may also be an expected decline in developmental indices with certain populations of handicapped children, such as Down syndrome children, who often do not maintain initial rates of development (Fewell & Sandall, 1986). When this effect is seen in the evaluation data it may also reflect unfairly on the program. All of these measures may inaccurately depict the efficacy of an early intervention program, either evaluating child progress too high or too low. Clearly, additional indices of progress need to be used.

Child progress is, of course, not the only factor that may be evaluated. It may also be appropriate to reassess family strengths and needs, looking first at issues targeted for intervention. It may be helpful to repeat measures used in the initial family assessment (see Chapter 6).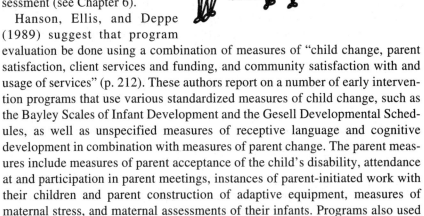

Hanson, Ellis, and Deppe (1989) suggest that program evaluation be done using a combination of measures of "child change, parent satisfaction, client services and funding, and community satisfaction with and usage of services" (p. 212). These authors report on a number of early intervention programs that use various standardized measures of child change, such as the Bayley Scales of Infant Development and the Gesell Developmental Schedules, as well as unspecified measures of receptive language and cognitive development in combination with measures of parent change. The parent measures include measures of parent acceptance of the child's disability, attendance at and participation in parent meetings, instances of parent-initiated work with their children and parent construction of adaptive equipment, measures of maternal stress, and maternal assessments of their infants. Programs also used more standard tools, such as the Home Observation for Measurement of the Environment (HOME) scale (Bradley & Caldwell, 1978), the Parent Behavior Progression (PBP) (Bromwich, 1981), and the Nursing Child Assessment Teaching Scale (NCAT) (Barnard, 1978).

Slentz, Walker, and Bricker (1989) report on a program that was designed to involve parents in a number of different roles through a parent-to-parent training sequence. The focus of program evaluation for this approach was, therefore, to measure the impact on parents of their involvement in the program. This was accomplished by measuring parent participation, parent attitudes about their competence as parents of children with special needs, parent satisfaction with the program, and training impact from sources such as program documents, self-report measures (the Parental Self-Appraisal Inventory [Carter & Macy, 1978] and the Parent Survey [Roberts, undated]), and supervisor report.

In addition to these outcome measures, Campbell (1989a) suggests a form of evaluation that looks at the process of intervention. Campbell suggests that a list of "quality indicators" be developed from literature which describes "best practices" for intervention with young children, selecting those that are deemed important by administrators, staff, and families, and that are consistent with the program philosophy. These quality indicators may be in the form of statements with which the respondent can agree or disagree, e.g., "Staff communicate concerns about children to families in a positive manner," and "Staff ask families for information that help children be more active participants in class-room activities" (p. 14). Using the indicators, evaluators—who may be con-sumers (parents), staff, funding agency representatives, administrators, or inde-pendent evaluators—complete checklists as they do direct observations of the program, reviews of records, and interviews with various constituency groups to assess perceptions of services.

The issue of whether the program is successful in its attempt to be family centered has also been addressed by a number of programs. Some programs have dealt with the issue by using family-completed questionnaires that are designed to evaluate the family centeredness of the program, the family's perception of the program and its staff members, and their general satisfaction with the program. An example of such a rating scale is the Family-Centered Program Rating Scale: Parents' Scale (Murphy, Lee, Turbiville, Turnbull, & Summers, 1991) (see Appendix 10-A). The rating scale is also available in a Spanish language version.

Similarly, professionals have been encouraged by some to complete ques-tionnaires that assess the extent to which program policies and practices reflect a family-centered approach. One instrument that has been designed for this purpose is *Brass Tacks: A Self-Rating of Family-Centered Practices in Early Intervention* (McWilliam & Winton, 1991). *Brass Tacks* is divided into two parts. Part 1 is designed to be used by any and all program personnel and deals with global policies and procedures. Part 2 is for use by the staff members who have regular contact with families and addresses their specific interactions with these families. Both of the scales are divided into four sections: (1) first en-counters with families; (2) identifying goals for intervention (child and family assessment); (3) intervention planning for children and families; and (4) day-to-day service provision. Exhibit 10-1 contains sample questions from each of these scales.

Another comparable, but much shorter, instrument has been developed for completion by families and staff together. This program checklist (Campbell, 1989a) is designed to help programs to develop family-centered practices and policies (see Appendix 10-B).

Benefits to the community may be assessed by gathering data from some of its social institutions (by sampling public opinion and information formally or informally) or by longitudinally tracking outcomes for a group of children

Exhibit 10-1 Examples of Brass Tacks Questions

Part 1	Part 2
First Encounters with Families	
Do you ask other agencies and professionals to encourage parents themselves to make the referral to your program (i.e., parents make first phone call or write a letter)?	Do you give parents enough information to allow them to plan or prepare for the first meeting with professionals from your program?
Identifying Goals for Intervention	
Do you tell parents exactly who will have access to the information they provide and how the information will be used (i.e., informed consent and confidentiality)?	Do you have an understanding of the culture and value system of the families you serve? Can you accept their values, even when they are in conflict with your own?
Intervention Planning for Children and Families	
Do you offer parents the opportunity to be present at all discussions regarding intervention planning for their children and themselves?	Do you ask parents what they see as priority areas for intervention (what to work on with their child) before offering your own opinion?
Day-to-Day Service Provision	
Do you offer services at times that are convenient for families (parents have choices and make decisions)?	Do you encourage parents to determine the agenda (e.g., purpose, activities) for each home or clinic visit?

Source: From *Brass Tacks: A Self-Rating of Family-Centered Practices in Early Intervention* by P. McWilliam and P. Winton, 1991, Chapel Hill, NC: Frank Porter Graham Child Development Center, University of North Carolina at Chapel Hill.

through its school system. Measurable changes may be shown in decreased enrollment in special education classes, decreased costs of educational services, and long-term gains in increased employability and productivity, and/or decreased delinquency in program graduates. Or a cost-benefit analysis might be done to ascertain the cost of early intervention versus later special education for the same subjects (Barnett & Escobar, 1989).

Another issue concerning evaluation is when it should be done. Mori (1983) recommends that an evaluation plan be developed as part of the initial planning of an early intervention program. Thus, program evaluation becomes an ongoing process that is less distracting and difficult for the staff and clients. In addition, we must consider whether we are concerned with immediate outcomes or long-term effects. It has been implied that there is value in looking at both short-term and long-term effects of program interventions. We are certainly hopeful that our interventions have a measurable and lasting impact on child and family well-being, but any immediate positive effects, even if their long-term effects cannot be proven, seem valuable.

Bailey and Simeonsson (1988) suggest that program evaluators must also consider the interpretability of the information gathered. Questions to be asked include: (1) Can we attribute the changes (or lack of changes) to the intervention provided rather than to maturation, history, or familiarity with the test situation? and (2) Are the changes relevant and significant? Awareness of the question of attribution will help us to realistically assess our impact by considering other factors that might contribute to the apparent success or failure of the program. The second question may best be addressed by considering parent satisfaction.

CONCLUSION

In summary, program evaluation requires a number of different strategies for looking at the various areas of impact that are possible results of family-centered early intervention. Perhaps the most cogent source of evaluation is family satisfaction with the program. If families feel that they have been supported in their efforts to provide the best possible environment for child development, the program has had a positive impact.

Appendix 10-A

Family-Centered Program Rating Scale: Parents' Scale

Note: Potential users are urged to use the *Family-Centered Program Rating Scale* only with full knowledge of its rationale, psychometric properties, and instructions for scoring and interpretation. This information is available in the User's Manual, which may be obtained from: The University of Kansas, Beach Center on Families and Disability, Schiefelbusch Institute for Life Span Studies, 3111 Haworth, Lawrence, KS 66045.

Source: From *Family-Centered Program Rating Scale: Parents' Scale* by D.L. Murphy, I.M. Lee, V. Turbiville, A.P. Turnbull, and J.A. Summers, 1991, Lawrence, KS: Beach Center on Families and Disability, University of Kansas. Reprinted with permission.

FAMILY-CENTERED PROGRAM RATING SCALE

Parents' Scale

There are lots of different ways programs can serve families of young children with special needs. Which ways are important to you? How well do you think this program is doing? Your response to these questions will help us evaluate this program and plan improvements.

Directions: Each statement on this rating scale finishes a sentence which begins with the words at the top of the section. For example, statements in the first section begin with:

IN THIS PROGRAM . . .

All of the statements in the first section finish this sentence. There are four sections; each section has a different beginning. Read each statement and mark it two times:

1 Tell how well your program is doing on each item. Circle the letters that most closely tell us your opinion about how your program is doing.

P = **P**oor
OK = **O**kay
G = **G**ood
E = **E**xcellent

2 Tell how important the item is to you, personally. Circle the letters that most closely tell us how important this item is to you.

NI = **N**ot Important
SI = **S**omewhat **I**mportant
I = **I**mportant
VI = **V**ery **I**mportant

Start Here   **1**   **2**

A. IN THIS PROGRAM . . .

	1	2
1. meetings with my family are scheduled when and where they are most convenient for us.	P OK G E	NI SI I VI
2. the information staff members give my family helps us make decision about our child.	P OK G E	NI SI I VI
3. someone on the staff can help my family get services from other agencies.	P OK G E	NI SI I VI
4. services can change quickly when my family's or child's needs change.	P OK G E	NI SI I VI

	How well does your program do this? P = **P**oor OK = **O**kay G = **G**ood E = **E**xcellent	How important is this to you? NI = **N**ot Important SI = **S**omewhat Important I = **I**mportant VI = **V**ery Important

IN THIS PROGRAM . . .

5. services are planned with my family's transportation and scheduling needs in mind.

P OK G E   NI SI I VI

6. someone on the staff can help my family communicate with all the other professionals serving us and our child.

P OK G E   NI SI I VI

7. the program administrator makes my family feel comfortable when we have questions or complaints.

P OK G E   NI SI I VI

8. the IEP, or IFSP (Individualized Family Service Plan), is used as a "plan of action."

P OK G E   NI SI I VI

9. there is a comfortable way to work out disagreements between families and staff members.

P OK G E   NI SI I VI

B. THE PROGRAM . . .

10. helps my family when we want information about jobs, money, counseling, housing, or other basic family needs.

P OK G E   NI SI I VI

11. gives the other children in my family support and information about their brother's or sister's disability.

P OK G E   NI SI I VI

12. gives us information on how to meet other families of children with similar needs.

P OK G E   NI SI I VI

13. offers special times for fathers to talk with other fathers and with the staff.

P OK G E   NI SI I VI

How well does your program do this?	How important is this to you?
P = **P**oor	NI = **N**ot Important
OK = **O**kay	SI = **S**omewhat Important
G = **G**ood	I = **I**mportant
E = **E**xcellent	VI = **V**ery Important

THE PROGRAM . . .

14. offers information in a variety of ways (written, videotape, cassette tape, workshop, etc.).

P OK G E   NI SI I VI

15. helps my family expect good things in the future for ourselves and our children.

P OK G E   NI SI I VI

C. STAFF MEMBERS . . .

16. are available to go to doctors or other service providers with my family to help ask questions, sort out information, and decide on services.

P OK G E   NI SI I VI

17. help my family learn how to teach our child special skills.

P OK G E   NI SI I VI

18. give information to help my family explain our child's needs to friends and other family members.

P OK G E   NI SI I VI

19. help my family plan for the future.

P OK G E   NI SI I VI

20. don't ask my family about personal matters unless it is necessary.

P OK G E   NI SI I VI

21. respect whatever level of involvement my family chooses in making decisions.

P OK G E   NI SI I VI

22. don't rusk my family to make changes.

P OK G E   NI SI I VI

23. help my family feel we can make a positive difference in our child's life.

P OK G E   NI SI I VI

24. give my family time to talk about our experiences and things that are important to us.

P OK G E   NI SI I VI

	How well does your program do this? P = **P**oor OK = **O**kay G = **G**ood E = **E**xcellent	How important is this to you? NI = **N**ot Important SI = **S**omewhat Important I = **I**mportant VI = **V**ery Important

STAFF MEMBERS . . .

25. are honest with my family.

P OK G E   NI SI I VI

26. create ways for my family to be involved in making decisions about services.

P OK G E   NI SI I VI

27. give my family clear and complete information about our child's disability.

P OK G E   NI SI I VI

28. tell my family what they have learned right after our child's evaluation.

P OK G E   NI SI I VI

29. don't act rushed or in a hurry when they meet with me or my family.

P OK G E   NI SI I VI

30. don't ask my family to repeat information that is already on file.

P OK G E   NI SI I VI

31. don't try to tell my family what we need or don't need.

P OK G E   NI SI I VI

32. help my family feel more confident about working with professionals.

P OK G E   NI SI I VI

33. give clear and complete information about families' rights.

P OK G E   NI SI I VI

34. give my family clear and complete information about available services.

P OK G E   NI SI I VI

35. help my family feel more comfortable when asking for help and support from friends and other family members.

P OK G E   NI SI I VI

36. regularly ask my family about how well the program is doing and what changes we might like to see.

P OK G E   NI SI I VI

37. offer to visit my family in our home.

P OK G E   NI SI I VI

38. offer ideas on how my family can have fun with our children.

P OK G E   NI SI I VI

39. treat my family as the true experts on our child when planning and providing services.

P OK G E   NI SI I VI

	How well does your program do this? P = **P**oor OK = **O**kay G = **G**ood E = **E**xcellent	How important is this to you? NI = **N**ot Important SI = **S**omewhat Important I = **I**mportant VI = **V**ery Important

STAFF MEMBERS . . .

40. give my family clear and complete explanations about our child. | P OK G E | NI SI I VI |

41. help my family learn how we can help our children feel good about themselves. | P OK G E | NI SI I VI |

42. don't overwhelm us with too much information. | P OK G E | NI SI I VI |

43. get to know my family and let us get to know them. | P OK G E | NI SI I VI |

44. help my family use problem-solving skills for making decisions about ourselves and our children. | P OK G E | NI SI I VI |

45. give information that helps my family with our children's everyday needs (feeding, clothing, playing, health care, safety, friendship, etc.). | P OK G E | NI SI I VI |

46. help my family see what we are doing well. | P OK G E | NI SI I VI |

47. respect differences among children, families, and families' way of life. | P OK G E | NI SI I VI |

48. ask my family's opinions and include us in the process of evaluating our child. | P OK G E | NI SI I VI |

49. are friendly and easy to talk to. | P OK G E | NI SI I VI |

50. help my family feel more confident that we are experts on our children. | P OK G E | NI SI I VI |

51. enjoy working with my family and child. | P OK G E | NI SI I VI |

52. help my family to have a normal life. | P OK G E | NI SI I VI |

53. explain how information about my family will be used. | P OK G E | NI SI I VI |

54. give my family information about how children usually grow and develop. | P OK G E | NI SI I VI |

	How well does your program do this? P = **P**oor OK = **O**kay G = **G**ood E = **E**xcellent	How important is this to you? NI = **N**ot **I**mportant SI = **S**omewhat **I**mportant I = **I**mportant VI = **V**ery **I**mportant

STAFF MEMBERS . . .

55. help my family see the goods things we are doing to meet our child's needs.

P OK G E   NI SI I VI

56. consider my family's strengths and needs when planning ways to meet our child's needs.

P OK G E   NI SI I VI

D. MY FAMILY . . .

57. is included in all meetings about us and our child.

P OK G E   NI SI I VI

58. receives complete copies of all reports about us and our child.

P OK G E   NI SI I VI

59. is an important part of the team when our IEP, or IFSP (Individualized Family Service Plan), is developed, reviewed, or changed.

P OK G E   NI SI I VI

COMMENTS

What things about your child's program make it especially helpful and welcoming to your family?

_____
_____
_____

What are ways in which your child's program could be *more* helpful and welcoming to your family?

_____
_____
_____

Appendix 10-B

Where Does Your Early Intervention Program Stand?

AN EXERCISE FOR FAMILIES AND STAFF TO DO TOGETHER

Family-centered services are at the heart of the IFSP. Many states have not yet adopted procedures, guidelines, or formats for the IFSP. Most early intervention programs, nation-wide, are in the process of shifting the focus of services from the infant or child to the family. To get a head-start in the IFSP process, use the checklist below to assess your current services. Ask parents to complete the checklist, also. Then, develop a plan for becoming a family-centered program.

PROGRAM CHECKLIST

1. Families in our program generate all (or most) of the goals for their children.
   Always   Sometimes   Never

2. Our program provides the following services (please check).
   ☐ Parent-to Parent Support Groups
   ☐ Recreational Programs and Camps
   ☐ Respitality
   ☐ Equipment Loan or Exchange Programs
   ☐ Toy-Lending Libraries
   ☐ Sibling Support Programs
   ☐ Respite Care Programs
   ☐ Day Care and Babysitting Services
   ☐ Technology Assistance
   ☐ Parent Education

Source: From "Where Does Your Early Intervention Program Stand" by P. Campbell, 1989, *The Networker, 2,* p. 3. Copyright 1989 by United Cerebral Palsy Associations, Inc.

3. Our services are provided in as normal an environment as possible.
Always   Sometimes   Never

4. Our program receives information from local parent groups and shares information about our program with them.
Always   Sometimes   Never

5. Our program provides a variety of early intervention services for infants and young children.
Always   Sometimes   Never

6. We allow parents to speak first in team meetings.
Always   Sometimes   Never

7. Teachers and therapists identify appropriate goals for children. The importance of these goals are discussed with families.
Always   Sometimes   Never

8. Parents are members of our board or of a program advisory committee.
Always   Sometimes   Never

9. Our services for children center around needs for physical and occupational therapy or speech pathology.
Always   Sometimes   Never

10. Our services are based on parent-identified needs for their children.
Always   Sometimes   Never

11. We provide home- and center-based services.
Always   Sometimes   Never

12. Our focus in programming is on the infant or young child.
Always   Sometimes   Never

13. Our services promote the integration of the child and family within the community by not focusing services on children with handicaps.
Always   Sometimes   Never

14. Our services support the family in its role as primary caregiver by providing services identified by families as necessary to meet their needs.
Always   Sometimes   Never

15. Our program collaborates with other agencies in our community to provide comprehensive community-based services for families and their young children.
Always   Sometimes   Never

HOW DO YOU SCORE?

Give yourself 1 point for each family service checked in Question 1. Score 2 points for each time you marked ALWAYS, and 1 point for each SOMETIMES in all questions except #s 7, 9, and 12. For these, score a 2 for NEVER and a 1 for SOMETIMES. How does your program rate? Pat yourselves on the back if you scored between 24 and 38. You are really providing exemplary family-centered services. If your score is between 16 and 23, you are well on your way to focusing on the needs of families. A plan to rethink your program philosophy and shape current service goals and objectives will help you move toward effective programming for families if your score is below 16. Talk with the families who use your services. Listen to their perspectives, needs, and ideas. There is always room for improvement in any program—no matter how exemplary!!

Bibliography

Administration on Developmental Disabilities. (1988). *Mapping the future for children with special needs PL 99-457.* Iowa City: University of Iowa Press.

Ainsworth, M. (1967). *Infancy in Uganda: Infant care and the growth of love.* Baltimore: Johns Hopkins Press.

Ainsworth, M. (1985). Patterns of attachment. *The Clinical Psychologist,* Spring, 27-29.

Ainsworth, M. & Wittig, B. (1969). Attachment and exploratory behavior of one year olds in a strange situation. In B. Foss (Ed.), *Determinants of infant behavior* (Vol. 4). London: Methuen.

Alexander, R. (1987). Oral-motor treatment for infants and young children with cerebral palsy. *Seminars in Speech and Language, 8,* 87-100.

Alexander, R., Kroth, R., Simpson, R., & Poppelreiter, T. (1982). The parent role in special education. In R. McDowell, G. Adamson, & F. Woods (Eds.), *Teaching emotionally disturbed children.* Boston: Little, Brown.

Als, H., Lawhorn, G., Brown, E., Gibes, R., Duffy, F., & Blickman, J. (1986). Individualized behavioral and environmental care for the VLBW infant at high risk for bronchopulmonary dysplasia: NICU and developmental outcome. *Pediatrics, 78,* 1123-1132.

Alvy, K. (1981). *The enhancement of parenting: An analysis of parent training programs* (Grant Report-Volume 1). Rockville, MD: National Institute of Mental Health.

American Speech-Language-Hearing Association. (1988). Position statement on prevention of communication disorders. *ASHA, 30,* 90.

American Speech-Language-Hearing Association. (1990). Scope of practice, speech-language pathology and audiology. *ASHA, 32* (Suppl. 2), 1-2.

American Speech-Language-Hearing Foundation. (1989). *Speaking of prevention.* Rockville, MD: Author.

Anastasi, A. (1982). *Pyschological testing.* New York: Macmillan Publishing Co., Inc.

Anderson, N. (1991). Understanding cultural diversity. *American Journal of Speech-Language Pathology, 1,* 9-10.

Anderson, P. & Fenichel, E. (1989). *Serving culturally diverse families of infants and toddlers with disabilities.* Washington, DC: National Center for Clinical Infant Programs.

Anderson, W., Beckett, S., Chitwood, D., Hayden, D., & Hitz, N. (1990). *Next steps: Planning for employment team training manual.* Alexandria, VA: Parent Educational Advocacy Training Center.

Andrews, G. & Ingham, R. (1971). Stuttering: Considerations in the evaluation of treatment. *British Journal of Disorders of Communication, 6,* 129-138.

Andrews, J. (Ed.). (1986). The family as the context for change: Language habilitation. *Seminars in Speech and Language, 7.*

Andrews, J. & Andrews, M. (1990). *Family based treatment in communicative disorders—a systemic approach.* Sandwich, IL: Janelle Publications.

Andrews, J., Andrews, M., & Shearer, W. (1989). Parents' attitudes toward family involvement in speech-language services. *Language, Speech, and Hearing Services in the Schools, 4,* 391-399.

ASHA Committee on Language Subcommittee on Speech-Language Pathology Service Delivery with Infants and Toddlers. (1989). Communication-based services for infants, toddlers, and their families. *ASHA, 31,* 32-34.

Association for the Care of Children's Health. (undated). Family-centered care: What does it mean? (Brochure). Washington, DC: Author.

Bailey, D. (1987). Collaborative goal-setting with families: Resolving differences in values and priorities for service. *Topics in Early Childhood Special Education, 7,* 59-71.

Bailey, D. (1991). Issues and perspectives on family assessment. *Infants and Young Children, 4,* 26-34.

Bailey, D. & Bricker, D. (1984). The efficacy of early intervention for severely handicapped infants and young children. *Topics in Early Childhood Education, 4,* 30-51.

Bailey, D. & Simeonsson, R. (1988). *Family assessment in early intervention.* Columbus, OH: Merrill Publishing Co.

Bailey, D. & Simeonsson, R. (1990). *The family needs survey.* Chapel Hill, NC: Frank Porter Graham Child Development Center.

Bailey, D. & Wolery, M. (1989). *Assessing infants and preschoolers with handicaps.* Columbus, OH: Merrill Publishing Co.

Barnard, K. (1978). *The nursing child assessment satellite training.* Seattle: University of Washington School of Nursing.

Barnard, K. (1984). Toward an era of family partnership. In National Center for Clinical Infant Programs (Ed.), *Equals in this partnership: Parents of disabled and at-risk infants and toddlers speak to professionals* (pp. 64-65). Washington, DC: Author.

Barnett, W. & Escobar, C. (1989). Understanding program costs. In C. Tingey (Ed.), *Implementing early intervention* (pp. 49-62). Baltimore: Brookes.

Baruth, L. & Huber, C. (1985). *Counseling and psychotherapy: Theoretical analysis and skills application.* Columbus, OH: Merrill Publishing Co.

Begly, S. (1991, Summer). Do you hear what I hear? *Newsweek* (Special Edition), pp. 12-14.

Benedek, T. (1965). *Mothering and nurturing.* Unpublished manuscript.

Berry, M. (1969). *Language disorders of children: The bases and diagnoses.* New York: Appleton-Century-Crofts.

Beukelman, D. (1986). Evaluation of the effectiveness of intervention programs. In S. Blackstone (Ed.), *Augmentative communication an introduction.* Rockville, MD: ASHA.

Blackman, J. (1986). *Warning signals: Basic criteria for tracking at-risk infants and toddlers.* Washington, DC: National Center for Clinical Infant Programs.

Bohanon, J. & Warren-Leubecker, A. (1989). Theoretical approaches to language acquisition. In J. B. Gleason (Ed.), *The development of language* (2nd ed.) (pp. 167-224). Columbus, OH: Merrill Publishing Co.

Bondurant, J., Romeo, D., & Kretschmer, R. (1983). Language behaviors of mothers of children with normal and delayed language. *Language Speech and Hearing Services in the Schools, 14,* 233-242.

Bowen, M. (1978). *Family therapy in clinical practice.* New York: Jason Aronson.

Bowlby, J. (1965). *Child care and the growth of love* (2nd ed.). Baltimore: Penguin Books.

Bowlby, J. (1969). *Attachment and loss. Volume I Attachment.* New York: Basic Books.

Bradley, R. & Caldwell, B. (1978). *Home observation for measurement of the environment inventory.* Little Rock: University of Arkansas at Little Rock.

Bradshaw, J. (1988). *Bradshaw on: the family—a revolutionary way of self-discovery.* Deerfield Beach, FL: Health Communications.

Brazelton, T.B. (1983). Foreword. In M. Klaus & J. Kennell (Eds.) *Bonding: The beginnings of parent-infant attachment* (pp. vii-x). New York: C.V. Mosby Co.

Brazelton, T.B. & Cramer, B. (1990). *The earliest relationship.* Reading, MA: Addison-Wesley Publishing Co., Inc.

Bricker, D. & Carlson, L. (1981). Issues in early language intervention. In R. Schiefelbusch & D. Bricker (Eds.), *Early language—aquisition and intervention* (pp. 477-515). Baltimore: University Park Press.

Briggs, C. (1986). *Learning how to ask: A sociolinguistic appraisal of the role of the interview in social science research.* Cambridge, MA: Cambridge University Press.

Briggs, M. (1991). Team development: Decision-making for early intervention. *Infant-Toddler Intervention: The Transdisciplinary Journal, 1,* 1-9.

Broen, P. (1972). The verbal environment of the language-learning child. *ASHA Monograph No. 17,* Washington, DC: ASHA.

Bromwich, R. (1976). Focus on maternal behavior in infant intervention. *American Journal of Orthopsychiatry, 46* (3), 439-446.

Bromwich, R. (1981). *Working with parents and infants.* Austin, TX: Pro-ed.

Bromwich, R., Khokha, E., Fust, L., Baxter, E., Burge, D., & Kass, E. (1981). Parent behavior progression. In R. Bromwich (Eds.), *Working with parents and infants* (Appendix A & B). Austin, TX: Pro-ed.

Bronfenbrenner, U. (1977). Toward an experimental ecology of human development. *American Psychologist, 32,* 513-531.

Brown, L. (1989, Spring). Let's do it right: A parent's eye view of PL 99-457. *The Networker, 2,* 4, 16.

Brown, R. (1973). *A first language.* Cambridge, MA: Harvard University Press.

Bruner, J. (1977). Early social interaction and language acquisition. In H. Schaffer (Ed.), *Studies in mother-infant interaction* (pp. 271-289). London: Academic Press.

Bruner, J. (1983). *Child's talk: Learning to use language.* New York: W.W. Norton & Co., Inc.

Campbell, P. (1989a). Quality indicators in early intervention: What makes a program of highest quality? *The Networker, 2,* 13-16.

Campbell, P. (1989b). Early intervention: Serving young children in integrated programs: A process of transition and change. *The Networker, 2,* 9-12.

Campbell, P. (1990, April). *Evaluation and assessment in early intervention for infants and toddlers.* Unpublished manuscript, Children's Hospital Medical Center of Akron, Akron, OH.

Campbell, P. (1990, May). *The individualized family service plan: A guide for families and early intervention professionals.* Unpublished manuscript, Family Child Learning Center, Tallmadge, OH.

Carter, J. & Macy, D. (1978). *Project kids study of parenting competency* (Report No. SP 78-105-52-08). Dallas, TX: Dallas Independent School District.

Catlett, C. (1991, November). *Building blocks: An early childhood education program for speech-language pathologists and audiologists.* Paper presented at ASHA Convention, Atlanta, GA.

Censullo, M., Bowler, R., Lester, B., & Brazelton, T. (1987). An instrument for the measurement of infant-adult synchrony. *Nursing Research, 36* (4), 244-248.

Chapman, R. (1979). Mother-child interaction in the second year of life. In R. Schiefelbusch & D. Bricker (Eds.), *Early language: Acquisition and intervention* (pp. 203-250). Baltimore: University Park Press.

Chapman, R. (1982). Issues in child language acquisition. In N. Lass, L. McReynolds, J. Northern, & D. Yoder (Eds.), *Speech, language, & hearing. Volume I Normal processes* (pp. 377-422). Philadelphia: W.B. Saunders Co.

Cheng, L. (1987). *Assessing Asian language performance: Guidelines for evaluating limited-English-proficient students.* Gaithersburg, MD: Aspen Publishers, Inc.

Chomsky, N. (1965). *Aspects of a theory of syntax.* Cambridge, MA: MIT Press.

Clark-Stewart, K. (1973). Interactions between mothers and their young children: Characteristics and consequences. *Monograph of the Society for Research in Child Development, 38,* 6-7.

Condon, W. & Sander, L. (1974). Neonate movement is synchronized with adult speech: Interactional participation and language acquisition. *Science, 183,* 99-101.

Conti-Ramsden, G. (1985). Mothers in dialogue with language-impaired children. *Topics in Language Disorders, 5,* 58-71.

Conti-Ramsden, G. & Friel-Patti, S. (1983). Mothers discourse adjustments to language-impaired children. *Journal of Speech & Hearing Disorders, 48,* 360-367.

Cooper, K. (1990, April 22). Headstart endures, making a difference. *The Washington Post,* pp. 1, 12.

Cormier, L. & Cormier, W. (1984). *Interviewing and helping skills for health professionals.* Boston: Jones & Bartlett.

Cornett, B. & Chabon, S. (1988). *The clinical practice of speech-language pathology.* Columbus, OH: Merrill Publishing Co.

Coufal, K. (1991, November). Teaming models for assessment and intervention with infants and young children (collaborative consultation). Paper presented at ASHA Convention, Atlanta, GA.

Crais, E. (1991). Moving from "parent involvement" to family-centered services. *American Journal of Speech-language Pathology, 1,* 5-8.

Crais, E. & Leonard, R. (1990). PL 99-457: Are speech-language pathologists prepared for the challenge? *ASHA, 32,* 57-61.

Crnic, K. & Leconte, J. (1986). Understanding sibling needs and influences. In R. Fewell & R. Vadasy (Eds.), *Families of handicapped children* (pp. 75-98). Austin, TX: Pro-Ed.

Cross, T. (1977). Mothers' speech adjustments: The contribution of selected child listener variables. In C. Snow & C. Ferguson (Eds.), *Talking to children* (pp. 151-183). Cambridge, MA: Cambridge University Press.

Cross, T. (1978). Mothers' speech and its association with rate of linguistic development in young children. In N. Waterson & C. Snow (Eds.), *The development of communication* (pp. 199-216). New York: John Wiley & Sons, Inc.

Cross, T. (1984). Habilitating the language-impaired child: Ideas from studies of parent-child interaction. *Topics in Language Disorders, 4,* 1-14.

Culatta, B. & Horn, D. (1981). Systematic modification of parental input to train language symbols. *LSHSS, 4,* 4-12.

Darling, R. (1983). Parent-prefessional interaction: The roots of misunderstanding. In M. Seligman (Ed.), *The family with a handicapped child—Understanding and treatment* (pp. 95-121). New York: Grune & Stratton.

Darling, R. (1988). Parent needs survey. In M. Seligman & R. Darling (Eds.), *Ordinary families, special children: A systems approach to childhood disability.* New York: Guilford Press.

Davis, P. & May, J. (1991). Involving fathers in early intervention and family support programs: Issues and strategies. *Children's Health Care, 20,* 87-92.

Deutsch, H. (1945). *The psychology of women. Volume II Motherhood.* New York: Grune & Stratton.

Dinno, N. (1977). Early recognition of infants at risk for developmental retardation. *Pediatric Clinics of North America, 24,* 633.

Dorris, M. (1989). *The broken cord.* New York: Harper & Row.

Dunst, C., Cooper, C., Weeldreyer, J., Snyder, K., & Chase, J. (1988). Family needs scale. In C. Dunst, C. Trivette, & A. Deal (Eds.), *Enabling and empowering families: Principles and guidelines for practice.* Cambridge, MA: Brookline Books.

Dunst, C., Jenkins, V., & Trivette, C. (1988). Family support scale. In C. Dunst, C. Trivette, & A. Deal (Eds.), *Enabling and empowering families: Principles and guidelines for practice.* Cambridge, MA: Brookline Books.

Dunst, C., Lowe, L., & Bartholomew, P. (1990). Contingent social responsiveness, family ecology, and infant communicative competence. *National Student Speech-Language-Hearing Association Journal, 17,* 39-49.

Dunst, C., Trivette, C., & Deal, A. (1988). *Enabling & empowering families: Principles & guidelines for practice.* Cambridge, MA: Brookline Books.

Duvall, E. (1971). *Family development* (4th ed.). Philadelphia: J.B. Lippincott Co.

Duvall, E. (1985). *Family development* (5th ed.). Philadelphia: J.B. Lippincott Co.

Ehly, S., Conoley, J., and Rosenthal, D. (1985). *Working with parents of exceptional children.* St. Louis, MO: Times Mirror/Mosby College Publishing.

Ensher, G. & Sparks, S. (Eds.). (1989). Early intervention: Infants, toddlers, & families. *Topics in Language Disorders, 10.*

Erikson, E. (1963). *Childhood and society.* New York: Norton.

Escalona, S. (1982). Babies at double hazard: Early development of infants at biologic and social risk. *Pediatrics, 70,* 670-675.

Eyeberg, S. & Matarazzo, R. (1980). Training parents as therapists: A comparison between individual parent-child interaction training and parent group didactic training. *Journal of Clinical Psychology, 36,* 492-499.

Fewell, R. (1986). A handicapped child in the family. In R. Fewell & P. Vadasy (Eds.), *Families of handicapped children* (pp. 3-34). Austin, TX: Pro-Ed.

Fewell, R. & Sandall, S. (1986). Developmental testing of handicapped infants: A measurement dilemma. *Topics in Early Childhood Special Education, 6,* 86-99.

Fewell, R. & Vadasy, P. (Eds.). (1986). *Families of handicapped children.* Austin, TX: Pro-Ed.

Fey, M. (1986). *Language intervention with young children.* San Diego, CA: College-Hill Press.

Final regulations, early intervention program for infants and toddlers with handicaps. (June 22, 1989). *Federal Register,* pp. 26306-26348.

Finn, D. & Vadasy, P. (1988). *Prioritizing family needs scale.* Unpublished manuscript, University of Washington, Experimental Education Unit, Seattle, WA.

Fitzgerald, M. & Karnes, D. (1987). A parent-implemented language model for at-risk and developmentally delayed preschool children. *Topics in Language Disorders, 7,* 31-46.

Foley, V. (1987). *An introduction to family therapy* (2nd ed.). New York: Grune & Stratton.

Food and Nutrition Service and Public Health Service. *Cross-cultural counseling: A guide for nutrition and health counselors (Fns-250).* Washington, DC: U.S. Department of Agriculture and U.S. Department of Health and Human Services.

Fraiberg, S. (1980). *Clinical studies in infant mental health.* New York: Basic Books.

Frassinelli, L., Superior, K., & Meyers, J. (1983). A consultation model for speech and language intervention. *ASHA, 25,* 25-30.

Gabel, H. & Kotsch, L. (1981). Extended families and young handicapped children. *Topics in Early Childhood Special Education, 1,* 29-35.

Gargiulo, R. (1984, Fall). Just suppose . . . parental reactions to the handicapped child. *Houghton Mifflin/Educators' Forum,* pp. 5-6.

Garrett, A. (1970). *Interviewing its principles and methods.* New York: Family Service Association of America.

Garvey, C. (1977). *Play.* Cambridge, MA: Harvard University Press.

Girolametto, L., Greenberg, J., and Manolson, H.A. (1986). Developing dialogue skills: The Hanen early language parent program. *Seminars in Speech and Language, 7,* 367-381.

Goode, W. (1982). *The family* (2nd ed.). Englewood Cliffs, NJ: Prentice-Hall, Inc.

Goodman, G. & Esterly, G. (1988). *The talk book.* Emmaus, PA: Rodale Press.

Gray, B. & Ryan, B. (1973). *A language program for the nonlanguage child.* Champaign, IL: Research Press.

Greenacre, P. (1971). *Emotional growth: Volume II.* New York: International Universities Press.

Greenfield, P. (1969). Who is dada? Some aspects of the semantic and phonological development of a child's first word. Unpublished paper, Research and Development Center in Early Childhood Ed., Syracuse University, Syracuse, NY.

Greenspan, S. & Greenspan, N. (1985). *First feelings.* New York: Penguin Books.

Greenspan, S. & Lieberman, A. (1980). Infants, mothers and their interaction: A quantitative clinical approach to developmental assessment. In S. Greenspan & G. Pollack (Eds.), *Course of life* (pp. 271-312). New York: International University Press.

Grossman, F. (1972). *Brothers and sisters of retarded children: An exploratory study.* Syracuse: Syracuse University Press.

Guitar, B., Kopff, H., Kilburg, G., & Conway, P. (1981, November). Parent verbal interactions and speech rate: A case study in stuttering. Paper presented at the ASHA Convention, Los Angeles.

Guitar, B., Kopff, H., Donahue-Kilburg, G., & Bond, L. (in press). Parent verbal interactions and speech rate: A case study in stuttering. *Journal of Speech and Hearing Research.*

Gullotta, T. (1987). Prevention's technology. *Journal of Primary Prevention, 8,* 4-24.

Halle, J., Albert, C., & Anderson, S. (1984). Natural environment language assessment and intervention with severely impaired preschoolers. *Topics in Early Childhood Special Education, 4,* 36-56.

Hanson, M., Ellis, L., & Deppe, J. (1989). Support for families during infancy. In G. Singer & L. Irvin (Eds.), *Support for caregiving families enabling positive adaptation to disability* (pp. 207-219). Baltimore: Paul H. Brookes.

Hanson, M., Lynch, E., & Wayman, K. (1990). Honoring the cultural diversity of families when gathering data. *Topics in Early Childhood Special Education, 10,* 112-131.

Hardy-Brown, K., Plomin, R., & DeFries, J. (1981). Genetic and environmental influences on the rate of communicative development in the first year of life. *Developmental Psychology, 20,* 244-260.

Harrison, D. & Alvy, K. (1982). *The context of black parenting.* Rockville, MD: National Institute of Mental Health.

Hart, B. & Rogers-Warren, A. (1978). The milieu approach to teaching language. In R. Schiefelbusch (Ed.), *Language intervention strategies* (pp. 193-236). Baltimore: University Park Press.

Havighurst, R. (1952). *Developmental tasks and education.* New York: David McKay Co.

Hays, D. (1989, May). Assessing infants and toddlers: A family focus. Information presented in an ASHA Videoconference, Rockville, MD: American Speech-Language-Hearing Association.

Healy, A. (1983). *The needs of children with disabilities: A comprehensive view.* Iowa City: University of Iowa Press.

Healy, A., Keesee, P., & Smith, B. (1985). *Early services for children with special needs: Transactions for family support.* Iowa City: University Hospital School.

Heath, S. (1982). Questioning at home and at school: A comparative study. In G. Spindler (Ed.), *Doing the ethnography of schooling: Educational anthropology in action.* New York: Holt, Rinehart & Winston, Inc.

Heath, S. (1983). *Ways with words.* Cambridge, MA: Cambridge University Press.

Hess, C., Sefton, K., & Landry, R. (1986). Sample size and type-token ratios for oral language of preschool children. *JSHR, 29,* 129-134.

Hetenyi, K. (1974, November). *Interactions between language-delayed children and their parents—A case study.* Paper presented at the American Speech and Hearing Association Convention, Las Vegas.

Hubbell, R. (1977). On facilitating spontaneous talking in young children. *Journal of Speech and Hearing Disorders, 42,* 216-231.

Hutinger, P. (1988). Linking screening, identification, and assessment with curriculum. In J. Gallagher, P. Hutinger, J. Jordan, & M. Karnes (Eds.), *Early childhood special education: Birth to three.* Reston, VA: Council for Exception Children.

Ivey, A. (1971). *Microcounseling: Innovations in interviewing training.* Springfield, IL: Charles C. Thomas.

Jaffe, M. (1989). Feeding at-risk infants and toddlers. *Topics in Language Disorders, 10,* 13-25.

Kagan, J. (1971). *Change and continuity in infancy.* New York: John Wiley & Sons, Inc.

Kagan, J. (1984). *The nature of the child.* New York: Basic Books.

Kaplan, L. (1978). *Oneness and separateness: From infant to individual.* New York: Simon & Schuster.

Kaplan-Sanoff, M., Parker, S., & Zuckerman, B. (1991). Poverty and early childhood development: What do we know, and what should we do? *Infants & Young Children, 4,* 68-76.

Kaufmann, R. & McGonigel, M. (1991). Identifying family concerns, priorities, and resources. In M. McGonigel, R. Kaufmann, & B. Johnson (Eds.), *Guidelines and recommended practices for the individualized family service plan* (2nd ed.) (pp. 47-55). Bethesda, MD: Association for the Care of Children's Health.

Kenkel, W. (1966). *The family in perspective* (2nd ed.). New York: Appleton-Century-Crofts.

Kenkel, W. (1977). *The family in perspective* (4th ed.). Santa Monica, CA: Goodyear Publishing Co.

Kilburg, G. (1980). *A critical review and evaluation of language assessment tools designed for use with children birth to three years old.* Doctoral dissertation, University of Pittsburgh, Pittsburgh, PA.

Kilburg, G. (1982). The assessment of emerging communication. *Communicative Disorders, 7,* 87-101.

Kilburg, G. (1985, November). *Changing parent-child interaction in language treatment: A case study.* Poster session presented at the ASHA Convention, Washington, DC.

Klaus, M. & Kennell, J. (1983). *Bonding: The beginning of parent-infant attachment.* St. Louis: C.V. Mosby Co.

Klein, M. & Briggs, M. (1986). *Observation of communicative interaction.* In Facilitating mother-infant communicative interactions in mothers of high-risk infants, *J. of Childhood Communication Disorders, 10* (2), 91-105.

Knobloch, H. & Pasamanick, B. (1974). *Gesell and Amatruda's developmental diagnosis.* New York: Harper & Row.

Kramer, S., McGonigel, M., & Kaufmann, R. (1991). In M. McGonigel, R. Kaufmann, & B. Johnson (Eds.), *Guidelines and recommended practices for the individualized family service plan* (2nd ed.) (pp. 57-66). Bethesda, MD: Association for the Care of Children's Health.

Kubler-Ross, E. (1969). *On death and dying.* New York: Bantam Books.

Kupfer, F. (1984). Severely and/or multiply disabled children. In *Equals in this partnership: parents of disabled and at-risk infants and toddlers speak to professionals.* Washington, DC: National Center for Clinical Infant Programs.

Lamb, M. (1983). Fathers of exceptional children. In M. Seligman (Ed.), *The family with a handicapped child* (pp. 125-146). New York: Grune & Stratton.

Lamb, M., Thompson, R., Gardner, W., Charnov, E., & Connell, J. (1985). *Infant-mother attachment: The origins and developmental significance of individual differences in strange situation behavior.* Hillsdale, NJ: Lawrence Erlbaum Association.

Lasky, E. & Klopp, K. (1982). Parent-child interactions in normal and language-disordered children. *Journal of Speech & Hearing Disorders, 47,* 7-18.

Leonard, L., Prutting, C., Perozzi, J., & Berkley, R. (1978). Nonstandardized approaches to the assessment of langauge behaviors. *ASHA, 20,* 371-379.

Leone, M. (1989, Spring). Early intervention or early interference? One family's experience. *The Networker, 2,* 5, 20.

Lewis, M. & Rosenblum, L. (Eds.). (1974). *The effect of the infant on its caregiver.* New York: John Wiley & Sons.

Lieven, E. (1984). Interactional style and children's language learning. *Topics in Language Disorders, 4,* 15-23.

Linder, T. (1990). *Transdisciplinary play-based assessment*. Baltimore: Brookes.

Linhart, S. (1990). *How to be a service coordinator for children birth through two who are at risk and their families*. Dayton, OH: The Ohio Head Start Association, Inc.

Lund, N. (1986). Family events and relationships: Implications for language assessment and intervention. *Seminars in Speech and Language, 7,* 415-431.

Luterman, D. (1984). *Counseling the communicatively disordered and their families*. Boston: Little, Brown & Co.

Luterman, D. (1991). *Counseling the communicatively disordered and their families* (2nd ed.). Austin, TX: Pro-Ed.

Lyon, S. & Lyon, G. (1980). Team functioning and staff development: A role release approach to providing integrated educational services for severely handicapped students. *Journal of the Association for the Severely Handicapped, 5,* 250-263.

MacDonald, J. (1978). *Oliver: Parent administered communication inventory*. Columbus, OH: Merrill Publishing Co.

MacDonald, J. (1989). *Becoming partners with children: From play to conversation*. San Antonio, TX: Special Press.

MacDonald, J. & Gillette, Y. (1984). Conversation engineering: A pragmatic approach to early social competence. *Seminars in Speech and Language, 5,* 171-183.

MacDonald, J. & Gillette, Y. (1989). *Ecoscales Manual*. San Antonio, TX: Special Press, Inc.

MacDonald, J. & Horstmeier, D. (1978). *Environmental language intervention program*. Columbus, OH: Merrill.

MacFarlane, J., Smith, D., & Garrow, D. (1978). The relationship between mother and neonate. In S. Kitzinger & J. Davis (Eds.), *The place of birth*. New York: Oxford University Press.

Mahler, M. (1968). *On human symbiosis and the vicissitudes of individuation*. New York: International Universities Press, Inc.

Mahler, M., Pine, F., & Bergman, A. (1975). *The psychological birth of the human infant*. New York: Basic Books.

Mahoney, G., Finger, I., & Powell, A. (1985). Maternal behavior rating scale. *American Journal of Mental Deficiency, 90,* 296-302.

Mahoney, G., Powell, A., & Finger, I. (1986). Maternal behavior rating scale. *Topics in Early Childhood Special Education, 6* (2), 44-56.

Manolson, A. (1985). *It takes two to talk*. Toronto: The Hanen Centre.

McCabe, A. (1987). *Language games to play with your child*. New York: Fawcett Columbine.

McCormick, L. & Schiefelbusch, R. (1990). *Early language intervention* (2nd ed.). Columbus, OH: Merrill Publishing Co.

McDade, H. & Simpson, M. (1984). Use of instruction, modeling, and videotape feedback to modify parent behavior: A strategy for facilitating language development in the home. *Seminars in Speech and Language, 5* (3), 229-240.

McDade, H. & Varnedoe, D. (1987). Training parents to be language facilitators. *Topics in Language Disorders, 7,* 19-30.

McGonigel, M., Kaufmann, R., & Johnson, B. (Eds.). (1991). *Guidelines and recommended practices for the individualized family service plan* (2nd ed.). Bethesda, MD: Association for the Care of Children's Health.

McGonigel, M. Kaufmann, R., & Hurth, J. (1991). The IFSP sequence. In M. McGonigel, R. Kaufmann, & B. Johnson, (Eds.), *Guidelines and recommended practices for the individualized family service plan* (2nd ed.) (pp. 15-28). Bethesda, MD: Association for the Care of Children's Health.

McLean, L. (1990). Communication development in the first two years of life: A transactional process. *Zero to Three, 11,* 13-19.

McLean, J. & Snyder-McLean, L. (1978). *A transactional approach to early language training: Derivation of a model system.* Columbus, OH: Merrill Publishing.

McWilliam, P. & Winton, P. (1991). *Brass Tacks: A self-rating of family-centered practices in early intervention.* Chapel Hill, NC: Frank Porter Graham Child Development Center, The University of North Carolina at Chapel Hill.

Mellody, P., Miller, A., & Miller, J. (1989). *Facing codependence.* New York: Harper Collins.

Menyuk, P., Liebergott, J., Schultz, M., Chesnick, M., & Ferrier, L. (1991). Patterns of early lexical and cognitive development in premature and full-term infants. *JSHR, 34,* 88-94.

The Merriam-Webster Dictionary. (1974). New York: G. & C. Merriam Co.

Meyer, D. (1986). Fathers of handicapped children. In R. Fewell & P. Vadasy (Eds.), *Families of handicapped children* (pp. 35-73). Austin, TX: Pro-Ed.

Miller, J. (1981). *Assessing language production in children.* Baltimore: University Park Press.

Miller, S., Wackman, D., Nunnally, E., & Saline, C. (1982). *Straight talk.* New York: Signet.

Minuchin, S. (1974). *Families and family therapy.* Cambridge, MA: Harvard University Press.

Mitchell, B. (Undated). *Test notebook 13.* New York: The Psychological Corp.

Mordock, J. (1979). The separation-individuation process and developmental disabilities. *Exceptional Children,* 176-184.

Mori, A. (1983). *Families of children with special needs.* Gaithersburg, MD: Aspen Publishers, Inc.

Moroney, R. (1981). Public social policy: Impact on families with handicapped children. In J. Paul (Ed.), *Understanding and working with parents of children with special needs.* New York: Holt, Rinehart, & Winston.

Morris, S. (1982). *Pre-speech assessment scale.* Clifton, NJ: J.A. Preston.

Murphy, D., Lee, I., Turbiville, V., Turnbull, A., & Summers, J. (1991). *Family-centered program rating scale: Parents' scale.* Lawrence, KS: Beach Center on Families and Disability, The University of Kansas.

National Center for Clinical Infant Programs. (1984). *Equals in this partnership: parents of disabled and at-risk infants and toddlers speak to professionals.* Washington, DC: Author.

National Center for Family-Centered Care. (1990). What is family-centered care? (Brochure). Washington, DC: Association for the Care of Children's Health.

Nelson, K. (1973). Structure and strategy in learning to talk. *Monographs of the Society for Research in Child Development, 38.*

The Networker, Vol. 2, No. 3. (Spring, 1989). Washington, DC: United Cerebral Palsy Associations.

Newport, E. (1976). Motherese: The speech of mothers to young children. In N. Castellan, D. Pisooni, & G. Potts (Eds.), *Cognitive theory* (Vol. 2). Hillsdale, NJ: Erlbaum.

Nichols, M. (1988). *The power of the family.* New York: Simon & Schuster.

Nock, S. (1987). *Sociology of the family.* Englewood Cliffs, NJ: Prentice-Hall, Inc.

Olson, S., Bates, J., & Bales, K. (1984). Mother infant interaction and the development of individual differences in children's cognitive competence. *Developmental Psychology, 20,* 166-179.

Owens, R. (1982). Diagnostic interaction survey. In *Program for the acquisition of language with the severely impaired.* San Antonio, TX: The Psychological Corporation.

Owens, R. (1988). *Language development: An introduction* (2nd ed.). Columbus, OH: Merrill Publishing Co.

Palfrey, J., Singer, J., Walker, D., & Butler, J. (1987). Early identification of children's special needs: A study of five metropolitan communities. *Journal of Pediatrics, 3,* 651.

Parke, R. & Tinsley, B. (1982). The early environment of the at-risk infant: Expanding the social context. In D. Bricker (Ed.), *Intervention with at-risk and handicapped infants* (pp. 153-177). Baltimore: University Park Press.

Parten, M. (1971). Social play among preschool children. In R. Herron & B. Sutton-Smith (Eds.), *Child's play* (pp. 83-95). New York: John Wiley & Sons, Inc.

Patton, M. (1980). *Qualitative evaluation methods.* Beverly Hills, CA: Sage Publications.

Price, P. (1983). A preliminary report on an investigation into mother-child verbal interaction strategies with mothers of young developmentally delayed children. *Australian Journal of Human Communication Disorders, 11,* 17-24.

Price-Bonham, S. & Addison, S. (1978). Families and mentally retarded children: Emphasis on the father. *The Family Coordinator, 27,* 221.

Public Law 99-457. (1986). *Education of the handicapped act amendments of 1986, Title I, Handicapped infants and toddlers.* Washington, DC: House Congressional Record.

Ramey, C. & Baker-Ward, L. (1982). Psychosocial retardation and the early experience paradigm. In D. Bricker (Ed.), *Interaction with at-risk and handicapped infants* (pp. 269-289). Baltimore: University Park Press.

Ramey, C., Beckman-Bell, P., & Gowen, J. (1980). Infant characteristics and infant-caregiver interactions. In J. Gallagher (Ed.), *New directions for exceptional children: Parents and families of handicapped children.*

Rees, R. (1984). *Parents as language therapists* (2nd ed.). San Diego, CA: College-Hill Press.

Reiss, I. (1971). *The family system in America.* New York: Holt, Rinehart & Winston, Inc.

Rice, M. (1989). Children's language acquisition. *American Psychologist, 44,* 149-156.

Ringler, M., Kennell, J., Jarvella, R., Navojosky, B., & Klaus, M. (1975). Mother-to-child speech at 2 years—Effects of early postnatal contact. *Journal of Pediatrics, 86,* 141-144.

Ringler, M., Trause, M., & Klaus, M. (1976). Mother's speech to her two-year-old, its effect on speech and language comprehension at 5 years. *Pediatric Research, 10,* 307.

Roberts, T. (undated). *Parent attitude assessment.* Tempe, AZ: Arizona State University.

Rodgers, C. (1951). *Client-centered therapy.* Boston: Houghton Mifflin Co.

Rodgers, R. (1962). *Improvements in the construction and analysis of family life cycle categories.* Kalamazoo, MI: Western Michigan University.

Rollin, W. (1987). *The psychology of communication disorders in individuals and their families.* Boston: College-Hill Press.

Rosenberg, S., Robinson, C., & Beckman, P. (1986). Measures of parent-infant interaction: An overview. *Topics in Early Childhood Special Education, 6* (2), 32-43.

Rossetti, L. (1986). *High-risk infants: Identification, assessment, and intervention.* Boston: College-Hill Press.

Rossetti, L. (1990). *Infant-toddler assessment: An interdisciplinary approach.* Boston: College-Hill Press.

Rossetti, L. (1991). Infant-toddler assessment: A clinical perspective. *Infant-Toddler Intervention: The Transdisciplinary Journal, 1,* 11-25.

Roth, F. & Spekman, N. (1984). Assessing the pragmatic abilities of children: Parts I & II. *JSHD, 49,* 2-17.

Russo, J. & Owens, R. (1982). The development of an objective observation tool for parent-child interaction. *JSHD, 47,* 165-173.

Sameroff, A. (1975). Early influence on development: Fact or fancy? *Merrill Palmer Quarterly, 21,* 267-294.

Sameroff, A. (1982). The environmental context of developmental disabilities. In D. Bricker (Ed.), *Intervention with at-risk and handicapped infants* (pp. 141-152). Baltimore: University Park Press.

Satir, V. (1972). *Peoplemaking.* Palo Alto, CA: Science and Behavior Books, Inc.

Satir, V. (1988). *The new peoplemaking.* Mountain View, CA: Science & Behavior Books, Inc.

Schrader, M. (Ed.). (1988). *Parent articles.* Tucson, AZ: Communication Skill Builders.

Scott, K. & Hogan, A. (1982). Methods for the identification of high risk and handicapped infants. In C. Ramsay & P. Trohanis (Eds.), *Finding and educating high risk and handicapped infants.* Baltimore: University Park Press.

Seibert, J., Hogan, A., & Mundy, P. (1982). Assessing interactional competencies: The early social-communication scales. *Infant Mental Health Journal, 3,* 244-258.

Shearer, D. & Shearer, M. (1976). The Portage project: A model for early childhood intervention. In T. Tjossem (Ed.), *Intervention strategies for high risk infants and young children* (pp. 335-350). Baltimore: University Park Press.

Shelton, T., Jeppson, E., & Johnson, B. (1989). *Family-centered care for children with special health care needs.* Washington, DC: Association for the Care of Children's Health.

Shieffelin, B. & Eisenberg, A. (1984). Cultural variation in children's conversations. In R. Schiefelbusch & J. Pickar (Eds.), *The acquisition of communicative competence* (pp. 377-420). Baltimore: University Park Press.

Siegel, L. (1982). Reproductive, perinatal, and environmental factors as predictors of the cognitive and language development of preterm and full-term infants. *Child Development, 53,* 963-973.

Simpson, R. (1982). *Conferencing parents of exceptional children.* Gaithersburg, MD: Aspen Publishers, Inc.

Singer, G. & Irwin, L. (Eds.). (1989). *Support for caregiving families.* Baltimore: Paul H. Brookes.

Slentz, K., Walker, B., & Bricker, D. (1989). Supporting parent involvement in early intervention a role-taking model. In G. Singer & L. Irvin (Eds.), *Support for caregiving families enabling positive adaptation to disability* (pp. 207-219). Baltimore: Paul H. Brookes.

Snow, C. (1984). Parent-child interaction and the development of communicative ability. In R. Schiefelbusch & J. Pickar (Eds.), *The acquisition of communicative competence* (pp. 69-107). Baltimore: University Park Press.

Sonnek, I. (1986). Grandparents and the extended family of handicapped children. In R. Fewell & P. Vadasy (Eds.), *Families of handicapped children* (pp. 99-120). Austin, TX: Pro-Ed.

Sparks, S. (1989). Family assessment. Presentation included in *Assessing infants and toddlers: A family focus* (Videoconference). Rockville, MD: ASHA.

Sparks, S., Clark, M., Erickson, R., & Oas, D. (1990). *Infants at risk for communication disorders: Professional's role in the home or center.* Tucson, AZ: Communication Skill Builders.

Spitz, R. (1945). Hospitalism: Genesis of psychiatric conditions in early childhood. *Psychoanalytic Study of the Child, 1,* 53-74.

Spitz, R. (1965). *The first year of life.* New York: International Universities Press.

Stern, D. (1985). *The interpersonal world of the infant. A view from psychoanalysis and developmental psychology.* New York: Basic Books.

Stewart, J. (1986). *Counseling parents of exceptional children* (2nd ed.). Columbus, OH: Charles E. Merrill.

Stickler, K. (1987). *Guide to analysis of language transcripts.* Eau Claire, WI: Thinking Publications.

Stone, J. & Olswang, L. (1989). The hidden challenge in counseling. *ASHA, 31,* 27-31.

Stonestreet, R., Johnston, R., & Acton, S. (1991). Guidelines for real partnerships with parents. *Infant-Toddler Intervention: The Transdisciplinary Journal, 1,* 37-46.

Summers, J., Turnbull, A., & Brotherson, M. (1985, December). Exercise: Social support, *Coping strategies for families with disabled children.*

Swope, S. & Liebergott, J. (1977). *Developmental language assessment and teaching.* Short course presented at the ASHA Convention, Chicago.

Taylor, O. (1987). Clinical practice as a social occasion. In the conference manual, *Communication disorders in multicultural populations.* Rockville, MD: American Speech-Language-Hearing Association.

Terrell, B., Schwartz, R., Prelock, P., & Messick, C. (1984). Symbolic play in normal and language-impaired children. *JSHR, 27,* 424-429.

Thacker, S. (1988, November). *Information on prevention from the Centers for Disease Control.* Paper presented at the Annual meeting of the Communication Disorders and Epidemiology Study Group, Boston, MA.

Thoman, E. (1981). Affective communication as the prelude and context for language learning. In R. Schiefelbusch & D. Bricker (Eds.), *Early language: Acquisition and intervention* (pp. 181-200). Baltimore: University Park Press.

Tiegerman, E. & Siperstein, M. (1984). Individual patterns of interaction in the mother-child dyad: Implications for parent intervention. *Topics in Language Disorders, 4,* 50-61.

Trivette, C., Deal, A., & Dunst, C. (1986). Family needs, sources of support, and professional roles: Critical elements of family systems assessment and intervention. *Diagnostique, 11,* 146-267.

Tronick, E. (1989). Emotions and emotional communication in infants. *American Psychologist, 44,* 112-119.

Trout, M. (1987). *Infant mental health: A psychotherapeutic model of intervention.* Champaign, IL: The Infant-Parent Institute.

Trout, M. & Foley, G. (1989). Working with families of handicapped infants and toddlers. *Topics in Language Disorders, 10,* 57-67.

Turnbull, A. (1991). Identifying children's strengths and needs. In M. McGonigel, R. Kaufman, & B. Johnson (Eds.), *Guidelines and recommended practices for the individualized family service plan* (2nd ed.) (pp. 39-46). Bethesda, MD: Association for the Care of Children's Health.

Turnbull, A. & Turnbull, H. (1986). *Families, professionals, and exceptionality: A special partnership.* Columbus, OH: Merrill Publishing Co.

Verny, T., & Kelly, J. (1981). *The secret life of the unborn child.* New York: Summit Books.

Vincent, J. (1979, March). A triadic systems model of infant integration into the family. In J. Vincent (Chair), *Learning to be a family.* Symposium presented at the biannual meeting of the Society for Research in Child Development, San Francisco.

Vincent, E. (1984). Family relationships. In *Equals in this partnership: Parents of disabled and at-risk infants and toddlers speak to professionals.* Washington, DC: National Center for Clinical Infant Programs.

Vohs, J. (1989). Recommendations for working with families and children with special needs from diverse cultures. And Organizational resources for understanding families from diverse cultures. In B. Hanft (Ed.), *Family-centered care—an early intervention resource manual* (p. 67 and pp. 69-74). Rockville, MD: The American Occupational Therapy Association.

Wanska, S., Bedrosian, J., & Pohlman, J. (1986). Effects of play materials on the topic performance of preschool children. *LSHSS, 17,* 152-159.

Warren, S. & Kaiser, A. (1986). Incidental language teaching: A critical review. *JSHD, 51,* 291-299.

Westby, C. (1980). Assessment of cognitive and language abilities through play. *LSHSS, 11,* 154-168.

Westby, C. (1987). Cultural differences affecting communicative development. In the conference manual, *Communication disorders in multicultural populations.* Rockville, MD: American Speech-Language-Hearing Association.

Westby, C. (1988, November). *Learning how to ask: Preparing to work with families.* Paper presented at the American Speech-Language-Hearing Association Convention, Boston, MA.

Wetherby, A., Yonclas, D., & Bryan, A. (1989). Communicative profiles of handicapped preschool children: Implications for early identification. *JSHR, 54,* 148-158.

Whitehurst, G., Novak, G., & Zorn, G. (1972). Delayed speech studied in the home. *Developmental Psychology, 7,* 169-177.

Wiener, H. (1988). *Talk with your child.* New York: Viking Press.

Wilcox, M. J. (1989). Delivering communication-based services to infants, toddlers, and their families: Approaches and models. *Topics in Language Disorders, 10,* 68-79.

Winnicott, D. (1958). *Collected papers: Through paedriatics to psychoanalysis.* New York: Basic Books.

Winton, P. (1988). Effective communication between parents and professionals. In D. Bailey & R. Simeonsson (Eds.), *Family assessment in early intervention* (pp. 207-228). Columbus, OH: Merrill Publishing Co.

Winton, P. & Bailey, D. (1990). Early intervention training related to family interviewing. *Topics in Early Childhood Special Education, 10,* 50-62.

Wood, P. (1980). Appreciating the consequences of disease: The classification of impairments, disabilities, and handicaps. *The WHO Chronicle, 34,* 376-380.

Wulbert, M., Inglis, S., Kriegsmann, E., & Mills, B. (1975). Language delay and associated mother-child interactions. *Developmental Psychology, 11,* 61-70.

Ylvisaker, M. (1981). *Infant communication questionnaire.* Unpublished paper, University of Pittsburgh, Pittsburgh, Pennsylvania.

Zelle, M. (1976). Early intervention: A panacea or an experiment? *American Journal of Maternal Child Nursing,* 343-349.

Zigler, E. & Berman, W. (1983). Discerning the future of early childhood intervention. *American Psychologist, 8,* 894-906.

Index